COLLABORATE

FOR SUCCESS!

Breakthrough Strategies for

Engaging Physicians, Nurses, and

Hospital Executives

COLLABORATE FOR SUCCESS!

Breakthrough Strategies for

Engaging Physicians, Nurses, and

Hospital Executives

Kenneth H. Cohn

Health Administration Press

ACHE Management Series

Your board, staff, or clients may also benefit from this book's insight. For more information on quantity discounts, contact the Health Administration Press Marketing Manager at (312) 424-9470.

Library of Congress Cataloging-in-Publication Data

Cohn, Kenneth H.
   Collaborate for success! : breakthrough strategies for engaging physicians, nurses, and hospital executives / Kenneth H. Cohn.
      p. cm.
   Includes bibliographical references (p.   ).
   ISBN-13: 978-1-56793-262-1
   ISBN-10: 1-56793-262-2
   1. Communication in medicine.   2. Hospital-physician relations.
   3. Hospitals—Administration.   4. Hospitals—Medicine staff.   I. Title.

   R118.C595 2006
   610.69'6—dc22

                                                    2006043619

The paper used in this publication meets the minimum requirements of American National Standard for Information Sciences—Permanence of Paper for Printed Library Materials, ANSI Z39. 48-1984.⊗™

Acquisitions manager: Audrey Kaufman; Project manager: Helen-Joy Lynerd; Cover designer: Robert Rush

Health Administration Press
A division of the
Foundation of the American College of Healthcare Executives
1 North Franklin Street, Suite 1700
Chicago, IL 60606-3424
(312) 424-2800

To the matriarchs of my family: my grandmother Regina Holland; my mother Ann Cohn; two cousins by marriage, Jimmie Holland and Joy Feldman; and my wife Diane Stowe-Cohn, who lent me their wisdom, tenacity, humor, and charm and encouraged me to make them my own.

Contents

Foreword

No one would argue that healthcare professionals are facing turbulent times. What is dismaying is the extent to which healthcare embodies a series of zero-sum transactions that pit providers against one another and put patients and their families in the middle. This diminishes service and the caring values that attracted many people to healthcare in the first place.

Nowhere is this deficiency more apparent than with patients suffering from chronic conditions, where lack of coordination of care and information leads to inefficient handoffs, suboptimal outcomes, and wasted money, time, and energy. This is a problem for individual patients and society.

The time to act is now. We cannot wait until local, state, or federal politicians come up with a solution to our fragmented healthcare non-system. Self-organization, a tenet of complexity science, postulates that new processes and structures can arise without being externally imposed.

Appealing to altruism is important but insufficient. Successful self-organization requires transcending short-term, zero-sum, win-lose transactions and substituting long-term partnerships, in which patients, families, physicians, nurses, hospitals, and employers all benefit.

If this process were simple, we would have done it already. The parties differ widely in their approaches, outlook, and experiences. Physicians have had no grounding that helps them understand the labyrinthine rules and regulations that govern hospitals. It may be similarly difficult for salaried healthcare executives to feel the angst of independent physicians who must use their time effectively and efficiently to pay their employees and meet their own families' needs. We must seek first to understand the opportunities and the stated and unstated needs of the constituencies.

Only by listening actively and carefully to one other and working together to expand and improve care can healthcare professionals collaborate effectively to serve their communities. Collaboration strengthens systems, decreases errors, and helps build a culture in which outstanding outcomes are the norm.

In his book, *Collaborate for Success! Breakthrough Strategies for Engaging Physicians, Nurses, and Hospital Executives*, Dr. Kenneth H. Cohn provides important thought leadership on the practical aspects of fostering and sustaining collaboration among healthcare professionals. Case studies in each chapter reveal examples of physicians, nurses, and hospital executives who have depersonalized differences and resolved conflicts to develop richer solutions to problems than would be achieved by any party acting alone.

This wide-ranging book on collaboration in healthcare discusses structured dialogue, the art of collaboration with abrasive professionals, new roles for hospitalists, crew resource management, socioeconomic issues relevant to collaboration, the Toyota Production System applied to healthcare, leadership development, evidence-based hospital design, the advantages of disease-based versus discipline-based care, proactive approaches to limit malpractice, blogs that sustain virtual practice communities, and academic medical center innovation.

I wholeheartedly encourage you to read these chapters and to apply at least one of the lessons to your institution in a timely manner.

—John Koster, M.D.
President and CEO
Providence Health and Services

Introduction

We need something that provides hope for healthcare workers. So many people are just holding on. They bring down the other people who have to work with them.

—*CEO of a rural New England hospital*

THE WORD "COLLABORATE" has two contexts. One context derives from the Latin *collabore*, to work together. A more negative context implies treasonous partnering with people who are not trustworthy, as in the phrase "collaborating with the enemy."

Doctors and hospital administrators have different training and perspectives that affect their approaches to patient care. They bring to mind conjoined bodies connected at the hip rather than at the head or the heart. Little in their training and professional culture prepares either party to adopt a truly collaborative framework. Moreover, the rapid pace of change and the time and energy required to collaborate effectively often leave them unsatisfied and feeling as though they are surrounded by enemies, with whom collaboration is perilous.

The purpose of this book is to discuss recent developments in healthcare collaboration. Effective collaboration is an underutilized method to boost revenues, cut expenses, improve outcomes, and use healthcare professionals' limited time more effectively. Collaboration also can promote patient and staff safety, satisfaction, and retention (IOM 2001).

Understanding the need for building a culture of collaboration requires a brief discussion of culture. Culture encompasses the beliefs, habits, attitudes, and assumptions that an organization develops to cope with problems (Duck 2001). It reflects a shared view of the world and of methods for problem solving proven to be effective in that world.

Effective executives make time to reflect on and shape organizational culture, because a strong culture allows leaders to delegate tasks, knowing that outcomes will remain consistently beneficial. Culture is dynamic, evolving with new experiences. It is assembled in stepwise fashion, one experience at a time. Ways that organizations can build an iterative culture of collaboration are discussed in the following chapters and case presentations:

- Chapter 1, "The Benefits of a Structured Dialogue Process in Fostering Collaboration," shows how a panel of practicing physicians analyzed care at their hospital and wrote a consensus report that established clinical priorities, refocused the hospital's business plan to provide better service to patients, improved physician-physician communication, and increased physician-administrator communication and collaboration.
- Chapter 2, "The Challenges and Opportunities of Collaborating with Creatively Abrasive Physicians," notes that getting along is a status-quo strategy. In contrast, partnering with abrasive but clinically outstanding physicians generated novel approaches and helped a healthcare institution improve care for its community and keep services from leaving the hospital.
- Chapter 3, "Maintaining Collaboration Between Hospitalists, the Hospital, and Primary Care Providers," reflects on the hospitalist movement and provides a checklist

of the actions necessary to improve communication among all three parties to maintain continuity of care, preserve loyalty of primary care providers, and facilitate retention of hospitalist physicians.

- Chapter 4, "Improving Communication, Collaboration, and Safety Using Crew Resource Management," explores ways that hospitals can learn from field-tested collaborative airline strategies to become safer and more reliable organizations.

- Chapter 5, "Socioeconomic Issues Affecting Healthcare Collaboration," analyzes long-term challenges that interfere with collaboration and suggests ways in which healthcare professionals and hospitals can survive and thrive in the future.

- Chapter 6, "Changing the Rules in Healthcare Collaboration Using Adaptive Design®," describes an evolution of the Toyota production method that allows frontline hospital workers to improve efficiency and decrease waste using a scientific, data-driven approach.

- Chapter 7, "Let's Do Something: A Cutting-Edge Collaboration Strategy," showcases the progress two nurses made using vision, leadership, and networking to establish a health careers consortium, overcome staff shortages, and achieve magnet status.

- Chapter 8, "Using Evidence-Based Design to Improve Collaboration, Clinical Outcomes, and Financial Performance," shows how design improvements can transform a healthcare setting, decrease patient and family stress, improve patient and staff safety, increase patient and employee satisfaction, and facilitate recruitment and retention.

- Chapter 9, "Collaborative Opportunities in Disease-Based Care" analyzes collaborative care in the sarcoma service of a cancer hospital to illustrate the benefits of disease-based care, including access to high-volume specialized services, participation in clinical trials, and improved survival.

- Chapter 10, "Taking a Proactive, Collaborative Approach to Malpractice Issues," acknowledges that effective risk management requires healthcare professionals to work in a more collaborative and proactive manner to avoid malpractice litigation and discusses seven developments that can decrease risk and improve outcomes.

- Chapter 11, "Building Community and Collaboration with Blogs," summarizes the role of Internet communication in creating virtual communities among physicians and administrators who see each other infrequently because of clinical demands, but nevertheless need to work together.
- Chapter 12, "Collaborative Leadership at Academic Medical Centers," explores the role of academic medical centers, a small but influential group of university hospitals. Academic medical centers can enhance collaboration among healthcare professionals through research, training, and the development of multidisciplinary innovative care models. In this chapter, department chiefs at a university hospital convinced surgeons to give up their elective block time and designate an operating room solely for emergencies, which greatly decreased the number of elective cases bumped because of emergencies and improved patient, family, and surgeon satisfaction.

The field-tested approaches discussed in this book involving structured dialogue, creative abrasion, crew resource management, adaptive design, leadership development, disease-based care, and Internet communication can improve healthcare professionals' ability to collaborate.

Effective collaboration creates a positive outlook that allows professionals with diverse backgrounds to develop new approaches based on shared vision rather than to play the role of victim (Ardagh and Wilber 2005). Collaboration strengthens social networks, which build trust, confer access to diverse skill sets, and nurture creative problem solving (Uzzi and Dunlap 2005). As such, collaboration can provide hope for healthcare professionals and help them to reconnect with values that attracted them to healthcare initially.

ACKNOWLEDGMENTS

I never expected to begin writing my second book within a month after *Better Communication for Better Care* was published. I owe a tremendous debt to colleagues who made time to review my first book and provide feedback on additional chapters that fit under the umbrella of improved collaboration. Those colleagues are now coauthors, and I could not have written this book without their patient mentoring on subjects in which I lacked their knowledge and experience. Additional friends and colleagues helped me improve the content and flow on short notice over the Christmas holidays. I thank: Ron Werft and Steve Fellows for helping with the creative abrasion chapter, Josh Hoffman for feedback on the hospitalists chapter, Tom Gagen for reviewing the socioeconomic issues chapter, John Roberts and Naida Grunden for their help with Adaptive Design®, Larry Maas for reviewing the hospital design chapter, Elin Sigurdson for improving the disease-based care chapter, Linda Haddad and Kathy Wire for their thoughtful suggestions regarding the malpractice chapter, Chip Souba for reviewing the chapter on academic medical centers, and especially my partner and mentor, Jim Dorsey, for reviewing every chapter before I sent them for additional outside reviews.

To my family, who put up with my genetically challenged attempts at multitasking projects, including providing locum tenens surgical coverage, consulting, writing a book, and studying for my board recertification exam in general surgery (which I passed to my great relief), thanks will never be sufficient. They took the burden of daily existence off my shoulders and allowed me to race ahead like a horse with blinders. I am also grateful to Augusta Horsey Nash, my partner in a mentoring program, who helped me be accountable to my daily goals, and to Sharon Hogan, who helped me write the book proposal.

Finally, I would like to thank the physicians and hospital executives across the country who inspired me and provided encouragement to write a book about changes in healthcare that give people hope. Working with you makes me proud to be a physician.

REFERENCES

Ardagh A., and K. Wilber. 2005. *The Translucent Revolution: How People Just Like You Are Waking Up and Changing the World*. Indianapolis, IN: New World Library.

Duck, J.D. 2001. *The Change Monster: The Human Forces That Fuel or Foil Corporate Transformation and Change*. New York: Crown Business.

Institute of Medicine and the Committee on Quality of Health Care in America (IOM). 2001. *Crossing the Quality Chasm: A New Health System for the 21st Century*. Washington D.C.: National Academies Press.

Uzzi, B., and S. Dunlap. 2005. "How to Build Your Network." *Harvard Business Review* 83 (12): 53–60.

CHAPTER 1

The Benefits of a Structured Dialogue Process in Fostering Collaboration

Kenneth H. Cohn, Andrew H. Nighswander, James L. Dorsey, and Robert B. Harrington

> A hospital CEO who thinks or acts like he has all the answers is like a doctor who self-treats his symptoms rather than seeking medical attention.
> —*California internist who participated in a structured dialogue process*

INTRODUCTION

Structured dialogue is a process that helps a group of practicing physicians articulate their collective, patient-centered self-interest (Cohn 2005). For example, structured dialogue can help physicians improve physician-physician communication, understand more fully the complexity of hospital operations, and articulate clinical priorities for their communities and their practices (Cohn, Gill, and Schwartz 2005).

Unlike hospital-centric change efforts, the structured dialogue process is led by a medical advisory panel (MAP) of high-performing, well-respected clinicians, who review and recommend clinical priorities based on presentations by the major clinical sections and departments. Contrary to the apprehensions of some hospital executives, the recommendations generally include performance improvements and minor expenditures that support these improvements, rather than a list of capital-intensive budget items. In return for giving physicians a say in clinical priority setting, the hospital is able to enlist physicians to attend meetings and outline their priorities. The benefits of effective physician-administrator dialogue are illustrated below.

CASE PRESENTATION

George's (a pseudonym) 6'2" height, deep voice, and impressive healthcare knowledge left no doubt about who was in command of his community teaching hospital. An industrial engineer by training, he used a precise, step-by-step approach, which his direct reports mirrored. He was the father figure that the managers looked up to. Yet today, his shoulders slumped, eyes stared at the ground, and voice trembled, "I have always been known as a turnaround CEO who came in, stopped the bleeding, and left five years later, with the hospital in much better shape than when I arrived. But now, I have been here eight years, and I just don't know what to do any more!"

He had tried the latest theories, including reengineering and rapid-sequence change processes, without success. Deficits increased, staffing decreased, and morale plummeted. With the encouragement of his senior vice president of marketing, who had witnessed a successful structured dialogue process at her previous job, and the approval of physician leaders, he appointed two talented and highly regarded physicians to be cochairs of a 13-member medical advisory panel. The co-chairs, not administration, picked the remaining members to represent outstanding medical staff practitioners from other departments (Figure 1.1).

The charge to the MAP was to engage physicians to analyze and recommend priorities to improve care for the community,

Figure 1.1: The Structured Dialogue Process

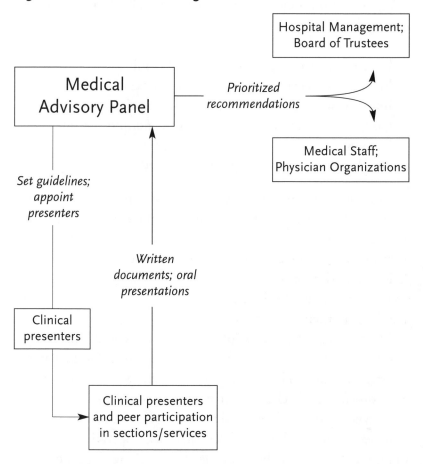

Reprinted with permission courtesy of the American College of Physician Executives. Cohn, 2002

physician-physician communication, and physician-administrator collaboration. Over the next six months, they heard recommendations from all major clinical areas to improve care for the community over the next three to five years. They chose a time span of three to five years to stretch participants' collective imagination and to encourage them to think about the future rather than the past. The panel's report listed approximately 100 recommendations from physician presenters that fell within four overarching themes:

1. Improve service to patients and their families
2. Enhance physician-physician communication
3. Implement clinical protocols in all major diagnostic-related groups to save money, limit variation, and improve quality and safety
4. Develop coordinated diagnostic and treatment centers

Although these recommendations may seem conventional to outsiders, the structured dialogue process represented the first time that the hospital administration had obtained a consensus report from its most talented clinicians. Furthermore, each recommendation derived from issues and opportunities raised in clinical section presentations. Previously, hospital leaders received feedback mainly from their "squeaky wheels."

Over the next two years, physicians, nurses, and administrators worked together to implement over 90 percent of the panel's recommendations. The remaining 10 percent were no longer relevant due to rapidly changing marketplace conditions. The structured dialogue process improved patient and employee satisfaction; increased surgical volume, market share, and operating margins; and groomed new medical staff leadership. The CEO now is a sought-after speaker at national seminars, explaining how collaboration with his practicing physicians was key to his hospital's recent turnaround.

CASE ANALYSIS

Hospitals of varying sizes (Table 1.1) have used the time-tested, structured dialogue process successfully by meeting the following three prerequisites:

1. Physicians and hospital executives must be interested in exploring how they can improve care for their community.
2. Practicing physicians must recognize the benefit of making time to prepare for and attend meetings based on their need to use their time better, increase practice revenues, improve processes of care, and/or leave a lasting legacy.
3. Hospital administrators and the hospital board must agree *a priori* to make every effort to implement the physicians' carefully thought-out recommendations, even if the physicians' suggestions represent a change in the hospital's business model.

During the structured dialogue process, physicians engage in face-to-face dialogue with one another and hospital leaders and learn to view their individual practices within a larger context. As the following quotations illustrate, the structured dialogue process is sufficiently flexible to be effective in a variety of settings regardless of size, geography, culture, and teaching status.

We ... came to realize that the stresses we faced were neither unique to our profession nor our community. What emerged was a viewpoint for the greater good, which greatly facilitated making difficult decisions and compromises. (Robinson and Skee 2004)
— *MAP cochair at 58-bed Southern hospital*

The MAP process works because, in the process of discovery, practicing physicians (whom the hospital does not employ) begin to think and act as owners.
— *CEO of 400-bed Northeastern hospital*

MAP members have had a unique opportunity to consult with their colleagues and take stock of current medical practice. It has become abundantly clear that we have lost touch with each other. Forces are being brought to bear which many of us have ignored or dismissed

Table 1.1: The Structured Dialogue Process at Hospitals of Varying Size

Hospital size	58-bed	200-bed	400-bed
Size of medical advisory panel	7	15	15
Reason for process	Improve communication and care processes	Improve communication and care processes	Improve communication and care processes
Catalyst for action	Threat of off-campus ambulatory surgery center (ASC) that would bankrupt hospital	Deteriorating revenue, market share, and physician loyalty	Need to engage physicians to plan for an uncertain future
Top recommendation	Site new ASC on campus	Improve IT services	Improve patient service
Outcome	• On-campus, joint-ventured ASC • Improved hospital and physician financial performance	•Improved processes in IT and Radiology •Improved market share in cardiovascular services, oncology, and surgery •Rebuilding of primary care network	•Business model changed from high-tech to more service-oriented approach •Clinical protocols established that cut variation and length of stay

because we have felt powerless to influence them. Our professional, ethical charge is to provide our services in the manner that is most beneficial to the welfare of our patients. We are now reminded that the hospital has the same responsibility. Our task is to work together to find solutions that will benefit all three—patient, physician, and hospital—and in so doing, gain strength from one another.

—Cochairs of 86-bed Western hospital

COMMON STEPS IN THE STRUCTURED DIALOGUE PROCESS

Over 30 hospitals and hospital systems in the United States have successfully undertaken a structured dialogue process by pursuing the following steps:

1. The hospital CEO and practicing physicians engage in a discussion of issues affecting care at their hospital.
2. Practicing physicians agree to participate in the structured dialogue process in return for assurance *a priori* that the CEO and the board will make every effort to implement the physicians' recommendations.
3. The CEO appoints two cochairs who are outstanding clinically, flexible in their outlook, and willing to invest time to improve care processes.
4. The cochairs pick a panel of 5 to 14 similarly talented physicians from different clinical areas.
5. The panel hears presentations from physicians in all major clinical areas after being briefed by administrators, including the CEO and vice presidents of finance, nursing, and information technology.
6. The chief medical and nursing officers attend MAP meetings to listen to the presentations and to provide information, as needed.

7. A talented administrative assistant assists with scheduling, room reservations, and other aspects of communication, for about five hours per week, on average, in the beginning of the process.
8. MAP members compile a data-driven, consensus-based report that outlines the top three to four major clinical initiatives (based on recommendations that presenters from multiple sections raise repeatedly) and lists the top five recommendations of every physician presenter, which they discuss with physician colleagues, administrators, and the board.
9. A joint task force of physicians, nurses, allied healthcare professionals, and administrators implement the major MAP recommendations in a timely fashion within two years.

KEY CONCEPTS

- The structured dialogue process reenergizes physician-physician communication and collaboration, resulting in specific ideas for improving care processes, the practice environment, and the institution's referral network; new net revenue flows from improved physician-physician and physician-hospital relationships and decreased outmigration.
- By giving physicians on the medical advisory panel timely information about hospital operations, the structured dialogue process enables physicians to understand and appreciate the complexities of operating a contemporary hospital, improves physician-hospital communication and collaboration, and serves as an effective training environment for new physician leaders.
- Active physician participation in the medical advisory panel that leads to timely and substantive changes in the practice

environment gives physicians a feeling that their time is well spent and makes it easier to find physicians willing to participate in joint physician-hospital task forces.

- The structured dialogue process can help rebuild physician loyalty to a hospital at a time when both primary care physicians and specialists are pursuing outpatient care opportunities.

REFERENCES

Cohn, K.H. 2005. *Better Communication for Better Care: Mastering Physician-Administrator Collaboration*, 4–5. Chicago: Health Administration Press.

Cohn, K.H. 2002. "The Structured Dialogue Process: A Successful Approach for Partnering with Physicians." *Click* [Online article; created 3/20/02.] www.acpe.org/Click

Cohn, K.H., S. Gill, and R. Schwartz. 2005. "Gaining Hospital Administrators' Attention: Ways to Improve Physician-Hospital Management Dialogue." *Surgery* 137 (2): 132–40.

Robinson. B., and J. Skee. 2004. "Picking Up the Pieces: Physicians Engage Each Other to Optimize Local Care." *Health Care Perspectives* (Summer): 9–10.

The Challenges and Opportunities of Collaborating with Creatively Abrasive Physicians

Kenneth H. Cohn, Thomas R. Allyn, and Robert Reid

> I would rather work with abrasive physicians than with board members.
>
> —*CEO of a large Western hospital*

INTRODUCTION

We tend to shun conflict in work settings. We find dealing with abrasive people difficult because they question our assumptions and make us feel defensive about our actions and values. In return, we label them as "not team players" and attribute qualities that allow us to downgrade their advice or ignore them. Abrasive professionals may indeed irritate, cause friction, and wear others down, keeping in line with the meaning of the Latin root *abradere*. However, they may also hold useful information that can keep a healthcare institution in touch with a dynamic market.

Conflict is inevitable in rapidly changing settings (Cohn and Allyn 2005). Surowiecki (2004) noted that diversity adds perspectives that would otherwise be missing and makes groups better at solving problems. Homogeneous, close-knit groups are often victims of "groupthink," as reflected in the Challenger shuttle explosion (Vaughan 1996). Hamel (2000) wrote that innovation is the defining competitive advantage of the twenty-first century. Independent thought increases the odds that an organization will make correct decisions and develop richer solutions in the face of ambiguity and paradox.

The purpose of this chapter is to point out the advantages of seeking out rather than avoiding creatively abrasive healthcare professionals who question assumptions and may not share hospital leaders' perspectives. The following case illustrates the journey of one of the authors, Thomas R. Allyn, a practicing physician who is evolving from avoiding hospital involvement to working actively with hospital leaders to improve patient care for his community.

CASE PRESENTATION

The Journey

I spend a great deal of my time working with dialysis patients in an outpatient setting. However, dealing with someone else's dialysis center, hiring practices, and policies and procedures grew ever more frustrating to my partner and me. We had no say in the operations of our local dialysis center. No matter how abrasive we became, we had no influence over the way the center was run. Therefore, we purchased a competing local dialysis center in 1988 to gain a say in operations, staffing, and policies and procedures. That purchase and subsequent control vastly simplified our lives.

My abrasiveness mirrored the abrasiveness of physicians who work at hospitals and cannot influence scheduling, staff, equipment, or policies sufficiently to predict procedure starting times, room turnover, and training of the staff assisting them. If you had told me 10 years ago that I would be a member of my hospital's strategic planning committee in 2005, I would have told you that you were crazy, since I never felt that any physician could really influence what a hospital was doing or where it was going.

In retrospect, my journey began late in 2002 when a medical colleague with whom I did my residency asked me to serve on what was called the medical advisory panel (MAP) to evaluate and recommend clinical priorities to improve care for our community. I was skeptical because I felt that the hospital had never gotten the service concept down and was incapable of fixing problems in a timely manner. Not wanting to commit to attending weekly 7:00 a.m. meetings for the next six months, I said that I would attend the first meeting and make a decision afterward. During a briefing before the first MAP meeting, I snarled at a consultant, "Don't waste my time!"

I quipped that, for this process to work, the hospital would have to undergo a cultural enema, in that decision-making processes and operations would have to become significantly more transparent, efficient, and timely for physicians to feel that their ideas mattered. I returned to subsequent meetings only because I was impressed by the quality of my fellow panel members and was willing to trust the commitment made by the board and CEO to give serious consideration to implementing the MAP recommendations.

I enjoyed the data-driven presentations, in which physicians from all major clinical areas discussed strengths, weaknesses, opportunities, and threats that they faced and recommended ways to improve care and to enhance physician-physician and physician-hospital communication. In addition, the MAP heard from the hospital CEO, directors of nursing and finance, and the chief information officer and obtained a perspective of the hospital and the complexity of its operations that we never had before.

During the presentations and the report writing that followed, the MAP thought openly and frankly about new programs and measures to improve operational efficiency without being encumbered by the hospital system's traditional business model and apparent "groupthink" approach to operations. We asked the hospital CFO to attend our meetings on eight different occasions to discuss ways that the hospital could improve its collection rate with different departments and sections. Our report, presented to the hospital board of directors in September 2003, represented the first time that the hospital had received a consensus report from practicing physicians about what the hospital should do in the future. Before, the process involved squeaky wheels pursuing individual agendas.

We evolved from a self-interested view of what the hospital should do for us as physicians to a more empowered view of how the hospital could employ limited resources to improve care for our community. Through the process of discovery, we began to think and act more as long-term partners and co-owners than short-term customers and renters. The MAP process allowed us to evolve beyond maintaining a level playing field for all physicians to leveraging hospital resources to meet community needs. That clinicians who prided themselves on patient care could come to consensus on long-term priorities gave the board and hospital administration the confidence to accept the MAP recommendations.

The Results

Although the report recommended the creation of an acute stroke center and improvement of throughput in the operating room and emergency department, which are in the process of implementation, subsequent accomplishments that occurred after the report writing are equally significant. The MAP has continued as an advisory body, meeting monthly with members of the administration and leaders of the medical executive committee and reporting to the board of directors annually. During the implementation phase, the MAP encouraged orthopedists to consolidate vendors, which resulted in a $1.4 million savings in 2004. In addition, the MAP is spearheading an ambitious program to limit sepsis mortality by accelerating identification of septic patients and antibiotic administration and taking measures to curtail ventilator-associated pneumonia.

The reason for my change in behavior stems from the feeling that I am making my time count and that we are truly making a difference. Previous service on hospital committees felt like wasted time because I did not feel that anyone with the power to do anything was listening, and nothing was implemented in a timely fashion. No one person seemed accountable, and the communication loop rarely was closed. There is no "we" in accountability (Patterson et al. 2005).

Now, after each MAP meeting, a scut list, similar to what I used during residency, contains the tasks, the one person responsible, and the timeline for action, all of which are reviewed at subsequent meetings. In creating such a list, we have built on previous successes and avoided death of innovation via the "slow no," or "let's study this some more...."

The MAP process has reinvigorated physician communication and patient care and made me realize the value of pooling ideas and talent. Previously, I did not realize how often we were talking at each other rather than to each other. Through the processes of dialogue, active listening, and discovery, I am dealing with some of the complexities in healthcare administration and have begun to think, work, and act more interdependently than independently.

CASE ANALYSIS

As outlined in Table 2.1, physicians have fundamental differences in outlook and training compared to hospital leaders (Cohn, Gill, and Schwartz 2005). While we acknowledge that neither group is homogeneous, Table 2.1 summarizes some differences to help depersonalize conflict and diminish divisive feelings that interfere with collaborative practice. In general, practicing physicians tend to employ a fast-paced decision-making style focused on individual patients. In contrast, administrators, who serve a wider constituency, tend to use a more collaborative and deliberate approach. When administrators are called upon to make more rapid decisions, it is often during an actual or impending crisis (Cohn, Araujo, amd Gill 2005).

An environment that encourages physicians to act as owners requires:

- Clearly delineated goal(s) that reflect active listening and a shared vision
- A strategic framework that encompasses physicians' customary ways of analyzing situations as reflected in Figure 2.1
- A timetable showcasing progress at regular intervals (no longer than monthly). Feelings of progress can be enhanced by using "chunking," or breaking up a large task into multiple small steps that convey sense of momentum and accomplishment.
- A next-steps task list with individual accountability for **outcomes,** not just processes
- Meticulous follow-up that demonstrates organizational commitment to closing the loop promptly and providing direct feedback to the physician who initiated an inquiry

Most physicians' are skeptical of the value of attending meetings because their income depends on seeing patients, they lose income when they are not providing direct patient care, and they feel that they rarely see evidence that their input influences decision making in a timely fashion. Physicians can bring focus to decision making with a fix-it-now approach, just as administrators can prevent costly errors by wanting to understand contingencies before making major decisions.

Many physicians underestimate the ambiguity and complexity that hospital leaders deal with daily until they (physicians) become actively involved in systematic clinical priority setting and build a shared community vision based on transparency and mutual respect. Few physicians understand the lack of job security faced by hospital leaders who serve at the pleasure of a board.

Table 2.1: Some Differences in Practice Environment Between Physicians and Healthcare Leaders

Environmental Variable	Physicians	Healthcare Leaders
Organizational scale	Generally small, < 25 employees	Large, > 100 employees
Sources of income	Consultations and procedures; Direct patient care	Largely salary, small variable component
Focus	Individual patient survival or improvement of symptoms	Organizational survival
Decision making	Rapid—based on individual judgment/experience, patient centered	Deliberate—based on consensus and review of multiple contingencies, patient and resource centered
Customary time horizon	Hours-days	Weeks-months
Timetable for change	Rapid, "yesterday"	Months to years (e.g., construction projects)
Gratification	Immediate, specific	Delayed, diffuse
Responsive to	Patients, families, colleagues	Patients, families, employees, physicians, community organizations, board of trustees

Figure 2.1: Contrasting Frameworks Used in General by Physicians and Hospital Leaders

Typical Physician Framework for Analyzing and Providing Patient Care
1. Take a history, gathering data efficiently and effectively using information technology and focused questioning
2. Analyze data and make a diagnosis that identifies all major problems
3. Start treatment, creating new or improved processes
4. Follow case closely and adjust as necessary, monitoring progress and modifying treatment where indicated
5. Expect to see effects of intervention quickly

Typical Administrative Framework for Analyzing Competitive Environment and Maintaining Organizational Survival
1. Identify macroeconomic trends including economic growth, interest rates, and global economic pressures
2. Note industry changes including federal, state, and local regulations, demographics, and impact of new technology
3. Brainstorm competitive response to changes and what will differentiate care at this institution
4. Assess customer needs and changes over time
5. Factor in relevant supplier issues
6. Focus on internal needs and changes over time

Two reasons that the MAP process takes longer than a weekend retreat are that it takes significant time for the MAP to review the recommendations of all major clinical areas and to evolve as a group in which each person becomes comfortable with others' perspectives, frameworks for analyzing data, and customary ways of converting data into information that improve patient care (Figure 2.1).

We do not suggest that improved communication will erase physicians' current frustration over increased workload and decreased reimbursement or hospital leaders' concerns over razor-thin clinical operating margins. However, both groups share a passion for caring for patients and a desire to improve clinical outcomes that can transcend differences in outlook and training.

Throughout this book, we present the ways that encouraging and depersonalizing creative abrasion and dealing with conflict in a collaborative manner can improve the practice environment, facilitate retention of productive employees, and increase net income for both groups.

KEY CONCEPTS

- Plenty of physicians are looking for ways to leverage their knowledge, experience, and energy to make a difference and leave a legacy.
- Hospital leaders can use several strategies to engage physicians as co-owners:
  1. Engage physicians in clinical priority setting and implement their recommendations in a timely fashion
  2. Create clear goal(s)
  3. Understand physicians' customary ways of analyzing situations
  4. Establish a timetable that shows progress at regular intervals
  5. Create a task list with accountability for outcomes
  6. Follow -up to make sure that someone has closed the loop

REFERENCES

Cohn K.H., and T.R. Allyn. 2005. "When Physicians Compete with the Hospital." *Better Communication for Better Care: Mastering Physician-Administrator Collaboration*, by K.H. Cohn, 17–23. Chicago: Health Administration Press.

Cohn, K.H., S. Gill, and R. Schwartz. 2005. "Gaining Hospital Administrators' Attention: Ways to Improve Physician-Hospital Management Dialogue." *Surgery* 137 (2): 132–40.

Cohn, K.H., M.D. Araujo, and L. Gill. 2005. "Appreciative Inquiry." *Better Communication for Better Care: Mastering Physician-Administrator Collaboration*, by K.H. Cohn, 24–29. Chicago: Health Administration Press.

Hamel, G. 2000. *Leading the Revolution*, 18. Boston: Harvard Business School Press.

Patterson, K., J. Grenny, R. McMillan, and A. Switzler. 2005. *Crucial Confrontations*. New York: McGraw Hill.

Surowiecki, J. 2004. *The Wisdom of Crowds: Why the Many Are Smarter Than the Few and How Collective Wisdom Shapes Business, Economies, Societies and Nations*. New York: Doubleday.

Vaughan, D. 1996. *The Challenger Launch Decision*. Chicago: University of Chicago Press.

Maintaining Collaboration Between Hospitalists, the Hospital, and Primary Care Providers

Kenneth H. Cohn, Daniel Litten,
and Thomas R. Allyn

When the hospitalists in my area discharge my patients from the hospital, they never call me, and the paperwork is always delayed, so when I try to resume my patients' outpatient care, I am flying blind.

—Thomas R. Allyn, nephrologist

When hospitalists first started working here, I initially thought it would be great, and it was for the first few years. Now the problem is that they've become overworked and bitter. They're always looking for us to send people home from the ED, or to get another service to admit them. Other times, they're annoyed if we don't have the complete workup done in the ED. Isn't that their job? The whole concept of facilitating hospital stays seems to have been lost. It just doesn't feel like we're on the same team any more."

—52-year-old Southern California ED physician

Other doctors and departments here still think "hospitalist" is equivalent to resident. It's not. I'm not here to be at the beck and call of every other physician. I'm here to see my patients and, truth be told, perform billable services. I don't want to see every patient in the hospital. I need to have a life, too.

—33-year-old Southern California hospitalist (Daniel Litten)

INTRODUCTION

Hospitalists are physicians who specialize in caring for inpatients, allowing internists and family practitioners to focus on their office practices. According to Freed (2004), hospitalists serve as physicians-of-record for inpatients, accepting handoffs of hospitalized patients from primary care physicians (PCPs) and returning patients to their PCPs at discharge. The term "hospitalist" was coined in 1996 (Wachter and Goldman); currently, approximately 8,000 hospitalists practice in the United States, with estimates that the total number of hospitalists will grow to 20,000 by 2010 (Williams 2004). The purpose of this chapter is to discuss the role of hospitalists in fostering a more collaborative hospital culture and the steps that need to be taken now to preserve the loyalty of PCPs who no longer set foot inside the hospital.

Why Hospitalists?

Although hospitalist care initially developed to allow PCPs to focus on outpatient care, it has provided important dividends to hospitals as well. Hospitalist care has been associated with a decrease in length of stay, excellent clinical outcomes, and increased nursing satisfaction (Auerbach et al. 2002, Meltzer et al. 2002). Hospitalists provide 24-hour attending physician coverage, which is a boon to aging clinicians for whom being up at night and seeing office patients the following day has become burdensome.

Hospitalists also care for patients admitted from the emergency department (ED) who do not have a private physician, which facilitates finding an admitting physician for patients who do not have a PCP. In addition, hospitalists play an integral part in the inpatient education of residents and medical students in teaching hospitals (Freed 2004). The work of hospitalists supports medical and surgical specialists by generating consultations and procedures based on pathology that hospitalists discover in the course of admission. For all of the above reasons, hospitalists can play a key role in improving healthcare collaboration.

THE ROLE OF HOSPITALISTS IN IMPROVING COLLABORATION

Improving Systems-Based Care

Hospitalists are comfortable with a systems approach to care in addition to satisfying individual doctor-patient expectations (Amin 2004). Hospitalists implement evidence-based practice guidelines and outcomes improvement measures, helping to coordinate team members and decrease variation in inpatient treatment. Hospital committees concerned with quality and safety note that a more concentrated presence of hospitalists compared to PCPs makes it easier to gain acceptance of new protocols and guidelines.

Maintaining Ties to PCPs

An aspect of hospitalist care that has received little attention so far is how to maintain the loyalty of outpatient physicians who no longer make rounds in the hospital. By their communication with PCPs, hospitalists could function as a hospital's ambassadors to busy generalists who have options in most cities to send patients to a variety of treatment settings. As discussed in Sidebar 3.1, a proactive, systematic approach is necessary to discover PCPs' information and communication needs, maintain links to outpatient physicians and their practice administrators, and measure and improve outcomes.

Sidebar 3.1: Ways to Keep PCPs Linked to the Hospital Once Hospitalists Care for Inpatients

1. Facilitate communication with PCPs regarding admitted patients
   - Fax the PCP an admission note with the hospitalist's name and cell phone number for every inpatient as soon as possible after dictation
2. Offer flexible services, customized to PCP needs, such as:
   - Admission of patients nights, weekends, and holidays for PCPs who want to assume care of their inpatients
   - Vacation coverage
   - Telephone coverage for outpatients who have questions
3. Maintain active, ongoing, personalized communication every 1 to 2 months, according to the schedule desired by PCPs regarding:
   - PCP needs, especially regarding clinical information on their patients
   - Hospital outcomes
   - Policies and processes in need of evaluation and improvement
   - Feedback on timetable for improvement efforts
4. Convene periodic lunches for practice administrators in similar specialties to make them feel important and included:
   - Provide them with a hotline, answered by a knowledgeable human voice rather than a machine, to report pressing problems with a single telephone call
   - Follow up (close the loop) in a timely fashion to make sure that problems are resolved
5. Track all contacts and maintain accurate, up-to-date lists of physician needs and preferences
6. Provide an opt-in, electronic system for keeping physicians' passwords current, so that they do not need to call in when they learn of their expiration
7. Provide continuing medical education for credit (CME) at times accessible to PCPs and their staffs
8. Use a variety of communication methods, including:
   - Internet-based chat rooms (e.g., weblogs, see Chapter 11)
   - Compact discs of CME programs that physicians can listen to in their cars if unable to attend sessions in person; list new services and other noteworthy items in 60-second welcoming message at beginning of CD

9. Facilitate provision of ancillary services
   - Rapid access, web-based scheduling of diagnostic studies to minimize telephone time
10. Use hospitalists as ambassadors to attend PCPs' staff meetings and work to improve the PCP-hospital interface
11. Consider financial collaboration projects:
    - Coinvestment in medical office buildings to allow PCPs to build equity
    - Alternatives to joint equity partnerships, such as participating bond investments, in which PCPs can coinvest with specialists without investors suffering dilution of returns

Overcoming Work-Related Challenges

Because of the intensity of hospitalists' work, hospitals may struggle with how to right-size the number of hospitalists to match demand and to keep hospitalists from burning out. Their work offers many of the challenges of residency without the aid of residents, except in academic centers and community teaching hospitals. However, even in academic centers and community teaching hospitals, recent legislation mandating an 80-hour resident workweek increases the likelihood that hospitalists will be called on to bridge coverage gaps.

Compensation alone will not prevent workforce burnout. Maintaining the quality of the practice environment by improving dialogue among healthcare professionals, providing adequate time off for family activities and continuing medical education, and responding in a timely fashion to hospitalists' suggestions for reform are key drivers of recruitment and retention (Sidebar 3.2).

Some hospitals have found that creating an electronic database of physician preferences that physicians can update allows

Sidebar 3.2: Hospitalist Recommendations to Improve Care

When hospitalists were asked formally to recommend changes to improve inpatient care, the following suggestions emerged:

1. Interdisciplinary patient rounds including physicians, charge nurse, floor nurses, case managers, physical therapists, pharmacists, and social workers
2. Outpatient clinics for unassigned patients who do not have a primary care provider
3. Expedited credentialing processes to alleviate long waits in high-turnover or scarce specialties, such as hospitalists
4. Creative strategies, such as hospital-employed specialists (e.g., general surgeons and orthopedic trauma surgeons) to maintain specialty support for inpatients (especially uninsured or underinsured patients) who do not have specialist coverage
5. Improved access to patient data through:
   - Adequate numbers of computers and peripheral devices in each patient care unit
   - Simplified sign-in procedures, so that access to radiology, laboratory, and specialized reports (e.g., cardiology procedures) requires only one password or biometric measurement
   - Internet access that allows physicians to check on patients from home or office settings
   - Hospitalist participation in task forces to improve patient flow throughout the hospital
6. Patient case manager availability on weekends and holidays to expedite discharges and optimize bed usage
7. Strategic alliances with palliative care units, such as hospices, to provide care for patients with terminal illnesses outside of acute-care patient settings
8. Improved communication between physicians, nurses, unit secretaries, phlebotomy teams, and laboratory technologists, so that truly urgent laboratory tests are ready within 60 minutes from the time that they are ordered
9. Assurance that staff who page physicians have access to and know the results of patient data, including vital signs, laboratory values, problem list, medication list, and allergies
10. Hospitalist participation at training sessions for new employees to orient staff to physician communication issues

allied healthcare professionals to learn physicians' expectations for treatment without needing to page them frequently. Another complementary approach is to track savings associated with hospitalist care and reinvest part of the savings in protected time for interested hospitalists to pursue clinical research interests, such as improvements in systems of care (Meltzer et al. 2002). Nevertheless, the hours and intensity of hospitalists' work are likely to result in higher turnover than for other types of physicians, and recruitment of hospitalists will likely become a recurrent activity.

Hospitalists are not homogeneous. They have different personalities, perspectives, and training. Their alignment with the hospital may depend on whether they are employees of a hospital, multispecialty clinic, or an independent group of hospitalists. Alignment may also vary with age and the importance of lifestyle outside the hospital, as reflected in the opening quotes. Complete alignment with others' values is an illusion. A more realistic long-term solution than expecting complete alignment is to participate in open, ongoing dialogue with physicians, nurses, and administrators to improve clinical outcomes in an atmosphere of empathic listening and mutual respect, as described in the case presentations below.

CASE PRESENTATION I

"You're kidding, right? You want me to see somebody because he's got a bump on his head?" Dr. Brian Jones (a pseudonym) was irate. As a hospitalist at a 290-bed community teaching hospital, he was already busy. Now, every day seemed to bring another unnecessary request for consultation from the inpatient psychiatry floor.

Tom, the charge nurse on the psychiatry floor, was also frustrated. He usually enjoyed his work, but lately felt like a dentist pulling teeth when seeking attention for his patients' medical problems. "All I know is the doctor wanted him seen. You can call her if you want to talk about it. I'm just following her order."

"Fine. I'll call her. But it's hard to believe this consult needed to be called at 8:00 p.m." Dr. Jones hung up, resigning himself to evaluating another anxious psychiatric admission. In the past week alone, he had been called to evaluate a 41-year-old woman with "rough skin," a 50-year-old man with chronic headache wanting to take his usual dose of Motrin, and a 63-year-old woman with irritable bowel syndrome, stable for the past 20 years.

In the past, PCPs had been willing to provide coverage for their patients during psychiatry admissions, but now felt too busy in the office to accept extra duties. Additionally, as PCPs became more comfortable with the hospitalists' presence, they referred more inpatient complaints to the hospitalists' attention.

Hospitalists did not welcome calls from the inpatient psychiatric service. Many felt they were being called simply to get a history and physical exam on the chart, with flimsy medical complaints being used to justify the consultation request. They considered the work to be uninteresting, involving chronic complaints, the antithesis of what had attracted hospitalists to inpatient care. To make matters worse, payers were now starting to deny reimbursement for hospitalists' care, deeming the diagnoses inadequate for an inpatient evaluation. A few hospitalists rebelled, refusing to set foot in the psychiatry wing.

The psychiatry nursing staff noticed the increasing difficulty of getting their patients' medical concerns addressed. The issue had arisen at several departmental meetings. As one nurse summarized to the psychiatrists, "What we have now is a non-system. You guys either have to start taking care of these issues yourselves or find someone else who will do it!" Physicians, nurses, and administrators discussed solutions, including hiring a dedicated internist or physician extender to cover the psychiatry floor. Both seemed too expensive and complicated, requiring a potentially lengthy recruiting effort and training time.

With the involvement of the medical staff office, a new idea emerged. The hospitalists already were well-versed in the system and provided excellent availability. The main problem was finding an incentive to make their duties more palatable. A solution emerged in which hospitalists would receive a daily stipend for psychiatry coverage that would include performing a full history and physical examination on all new admissions and providing follow-up care as needed. This solution ended reimbursement concerns and added predictability to hospitalists' workload, allowing them to know in advance when they would need time for psychiatric admissions.

Three months later, the psychiatric nursing staff felt relieved because the solution had ended confrontational calls with the hospitalists in which the nurses felt caught in the middle. Hospitalist coverage of the psychiatry floor had become a dependable service.

CASE PRESENTATION II

Richard Smith (a pseudonym), vice president at a 440-bed hospital, was frustrated. As a large tertiary-care facility surrounded by largely rural communities, his hospital's strategy rested on outside referrals for specialists, including cardiologists and orthopedic surgeons. The gradual closure and service reductions in smaller nearby hospitals had helped him achieve his goal. Unfortunately, now his hospital seemed to be its own impediment to further growth. Outside transfers to his hospital had been flat over the past six months.

In discussions with ED and specialist physicians, a repetitive concern arose: How can we accept transferred patients with fewer hassles? Many specialties were stretched to begin with, and few were eager to assume primary responsibility for new patients. Even pulmonary intensivists were hesitant to accept transfers without an internist to accept patients for the post–intensive care portion of the hospital stay. As a result, transfers were delayed for hours while the ED and specialist sought an available internist.

The initial answer had seemed obvious—require the hospitalist department to come up with its own system for accepting out-of-town transfers. Unfortunately, recent hospitalist-administration negotiations regarding protocol development and reimbursement of care for uninsured patients had caused several hospitalists to feel underappreciated. Hospitalists refused to take on another mandated responsibility. One hospitalist group threatened to stop providing ED coverage for unassigned patients who had no primary care physician, and the other saw half its physicians resign in a three-month period.

The growing, barely manageable workload was hospitalists' top concern. In response, the hospital agreed to provide locum tenens support and to sponsor a recruiting effort to attract and retain an adequate number of permanent hospitalists. Furthermore, hospitalists were guaranteed a minimum of Medicare reimbursement rates for out-of-town transfers.

With the new system in place, accepting transfers from outside facilities became a smoother process for the ED staff. Specialists and surgeons were able to focus on the required intervention and defer other medical problems to hospitalists. Outside facilities and referring physicians developed rapport with the hospitalists. Both recruitment and retention improved when the hospital offered support and gave hospitalists a voice in policy development.

CASE ANALYSIS

As both examples demonstrate, hospitalists can address a wide variety of bottlenecks and frustrations involved in inpatient care. A potential obstacle is that hospital goals and hospitalist goals are not always aligned. Effective dialogue is important for both sides to understand each other's needs and discuss their differences openly to create support for any changes to be made.

For a hospital to gain the most benefit from its hospitalists, hospitalists must be more than a stand-in for PCPs. By their nature, hospitalists are flexible in their duties and willing to take on different roles. Making lasting system improvements requires tactful communication to identify areas that the existing system has not addressed adequately. Furthermore, hospitalists' collaboration is necessary for the success of any new system requiring inpatient coverage. New policies affecting hospitalists may require offering additional financial incentives and meaningful input into hospital operations. These costs may be dwarfed by the efficiency the hospital gains from improving collaboration with hospitalists.

KEY CONCEPTS

- Hospitalists can function as ambassadors to primary care physicians (PCPs), increasing collaboration, satisfaction, and loyalty.
- Hospitalists can help improve systems of care, which can improve quality and safety outcomes.
- Hospitalists can maintain and improve resident and medical school education in academic centers and community teaching hospitals.
- Optimizing hospitalists' contributions requires their input into hospital policies, procedures, operations, and systems development.

REFERENCES

Amin, A.A. 2004. "Identifying Strategies to Improve Outcomes and Reduce Costs—A Role for the Hospitalist." *Current Opinion in Pulmonary Medicine* 10 (Suppl 1): S19–22.

Auerbach, A.D., R.M. Wachter, P. Katz, J. Showstack, and R.B. Baron. 2002. "Implementation of a Voluntary Hospitalist Service at a Community Teaching Hospital: Improved Clinical Efficiency and Patient Outcomes." *Annals of Internal Medicine* 137 (11): 859–65.

Freed, D.H. 2004. "Hospitalists: Evolution, Evidence, and Eventualities." *The Health Care Manager* 23 (3): 238–56.

Meltzer, D., W.G. Manning, J. Morrison, M.N. Shah, L. Jin, T. Guth, and W. Levinson. 2002. "Effect of Physician Experience on Costs and Outcomes on an Academic General Medical Service: Results of a Trial of Hospitalists." *Annals of Internal Medicine* 137 (11): 866–74.

Wachter, R.M., and L. Goldman. 1996. "The Emerging Role of Hospitalists in the American Health Care System. *New England Journal of Medicine* 335 (7): 514–17.

Williams, M.V. 2004. "The Future of Hospital Medicine: Evolution or Revolution?" *American Journal of Medicine* 117: (6) 446–50.

CHAPTER 4

Improving Communication, Collaboration, and Safety Using Crew Resource Management

Kenneth H. Cohn and Jack Barker

To improve productivity and safety, I started using an aviation-style team briefing prior to surgery. I wanted to identify team members, specify their roles, and spell out our expected outcome. So I wrote the names of everyone involved on the OR white board, including the maintenance lady that cleans my room, to make sure that everyone knew the members of my team. One of the surprise outcomes that occurred after I had initiated team briefings was a quicker turnaround time in my operating room. It was the first time that the cleaning lady had ever seen her name attached to a team.

—*New England Surgeon*

INTRODUCTION

The Institute of Medicine (IOM), Agency for Healthcare Research and Quality (AHRQ), and Joint Commission on Accreditation of Healthcare Organizations (JCAHO) have recommended applying aviation principles of crew resource management (CRM) to improve patient safety and clinical outcomes (Musson and Helmreich 2004). The theory behind team training and CRM is that complex systems break down not because of engineering flaws but because people operating within the system fail to interact in a manner that ensures efficient, safe outcomes (Healy, Barker, and Madonna 2006).

The modern aviation industry has been able to establish and maintain an unparalleled safety record. The risk of dying in an airline crash is less than 1 in 3,000,000, versus 1 in 200 from dying of a mishap on entering a United States hospital (Berwick and Leape 1999; Leape 1999). Aviation and healthcare are similar in that accidents typically result from a chain of human errors, referred to colloquially as "the holes in the Swiss cheese lining up" (Reason 2000). By breaking this error chain, airlines have been able to make air travel the safest mode of transportation. Reducing medical errors also can decrease the costs, estimated at $37.6 billion annually, of which preventable errors account for $17 billion annually in the United States (Kohn, Corrigan, and Donaldson 2000).

The purpose of this chapter is to highlight field-tested aviation safety processes that improve collaboration, reduce errors, and are transferable to healthcare settings.

What Is Crew Resource Management?

Crew resource management is a process for improving safety by enhancing skill sets in decision making, performance feedback, cross-checking and communication, creating and managing teams, recognizing adverse situations (red flags), and managing fatigue (Grogan et al. 2004, Kern 2001). Many aviation CRM principles are readily adaptable to healthcare. The cornerstone of improving collaboration lies in each person taking a proactive role to improve team performance, recognizing that everyone on the team has a leadership role.

Clinical excellence alone does not guarantee an outstanding outcome. Cardiac surgical teams that learned a new procedure most rapidly were the ones who created a safe environment for learning

(Edmondson, Bohmer, and Pisano 2001). Changing an organization's culture from blame to a shared sense of responsibility occurs by enhancing skills in several areas related to CRM. Programs vary according to institutional culture. There is no such thing as a universal CRM program.

CASE PRESENTATION

Leaders of a Northeastern otolaryngology department selected a CRM approach to improve communication and teamwork in their department of over 150 surgeons, nurses, audiologists, psychologists, office staff, and physician assistants. The metrics that they sought to improve included throughput, patient and worker satisfaction, and safety culture perception, measured by the AHRQ safety climate survey (AHRQ 2005). Everyone in the department completed the survey, which surveyed agreement with statements such as, "I would feel safe being treated here as a patient." Survey data provided a baseline measurement of the organization's safety culture. The survey was repeated at the end of program implementation to determine the efficacy of the interventions. Only 69 percent of the survey respondents initially viewed the safety climate in the department as positive.

Approximately 10 percent of the department was interviewed to identify core issues that surfaced in the survey data, such as teamwork challenges, disagreement on sedation procedures, and management of clinical protocol violations. Teams were observed so that training could be tailored to departmental strengths and weaknesses.

All personnel attended a one-day CRM seminar that explained basic error management, teamwork, and leadership concepts and that used role-play and discussion to reinforce these concepts. Participants used in-house case examples to demonstrate how to improve teamwork. One commented enthusiastically, "I have worked in healthcare for over 20 years and have never spent this much time with a surgeon … now I understand better my role in patient care and how to work more collaboratively with others on our team."

After the seminar, a senior surgeon exclaimed, "I have never seen a group of people in healthcare so enthusiastic over a training program." Over a period of several months, workshops provided information on communication, collaboration, leadership, workload management, and conflict resolution.

Trained observers watched teams in action and provided oral and written debriefs to enhance participants' ability to employ newly acquired skills. Selected participants took additional training to become resident CRM experts, nurture desired behaviors in their department, and begin a hospitalwide training program.

After approximately a year of CRM training, the percentage of survey participants who felt that their department had a positive safety climate increased from 69 percent to 91 percent. As a result of improved collaboration and service quality, patient volume increased from 17,000 to 18,355 in one year, resulting in a 30 percent increase in revenue. Referring physicians rated the department as one of the best services in the hospital, and practice administrators who were initially skeptical became advocates for extending the program.

CASE ANALYSIS

CRM training helps people feel more comfortable about intervening in patient safety matters despite perceived differences in status. An audiologist commented, "Before the CRM training, I would have minded my own business, but I overheard two anesthesiologists discussing dosage and realized they were about to overdose an infant. I decided to speak out as my CRM training taught me, and I know I saved that baby's life." The formal and informal mechanisms specified in the six steps of implementation below allow people to train and become confident in approaching patient care in a systematic way that heightens communication, improves teamwork, and reduces the risk of error.

Most programs begin after leaders attend conferences or read about CRM in the medical literature. For some institutions, a sentinel event provides the motivation to change, as with aviation during the previous century. Table 4.1 outlines the six phases of CRM training: organizational assessment, team training, targeted workshops, facilitated debriefs, coaching, and outcomes assessment, discussed below.

CRM Program Implementation

Phase 1. Organizational Assessment

The purpose of this phase is to understand the organizational culture, obtain buy-in from leaders and staff, and agree on metrics that define success, such as patient throughput, satisfaction scores, and clinical and financial outcomes. Participants answer the AHRQ safety perception questionnaire, as described in the case history. The data from questionnaires help define team issues that are unique to each organization. The organizational assessment phase is an opportunity to determine the organizational strengths and weaknesses that will influence the design of the next phase. Organizational assessment also allows leaders to gauge readiness to undergo cultural change.

Phase 2. CRM Team Training

The goal of this phase is to introduce the concepts of CRM and specific aviation safety tools, such as briefing, debriefing, and recognition and handling of adverse situations. All personnel participate in an interactive seminar that lasts approximately six hours, as outlined in Sidebar 4.1. Medical error studies and examples of

Table 4.1: Phases of Healthcare CRM Training

Phase	Month	Method	Learning Outcomes
1. Organizational Assessment	0–2	• Safety Climate Survey • Observations • Targeted interviews • Presentation of results	• Assess safety culture • Agree on metrics to determine efficacy • Identify personnel who will act as change agents • Determine readiness for CRM
2. CRM Team Training	2–4	Interactive seminar	Familiarize all personnel with CRM principles and tools
3. Targeted Workshops	3–5	Interactive workshops	Provide advanced training in CRM principles and tools
4. Facilitated Debriefs	6–8	Observations of teams and debriefs, two per department	Assess participants' progress
5. CRM Coaching	4–24	Individual coaching via phone and email	Equip change agents with knowledge and skills to continue the cultural change process
6. Outcomes Assessment	12	Safety Climate Survey analysis of designated metrics	Modify phases 2 to 5 based on outcomes

medical successes achieved through CRM help to overcome initial skepticism that CRM is a fad. The goal of having everyone present is to stimulate dialogue and reduce the influence of hierarchy in multidisciplinary processes that affect patient safety.

Phase 3. Targeted Workshops

In this phase, participants build on insights learned during the survey and seminar. The purpose of this phase is to continue the cultural change toward a more teamwork-oriented and safety-conscious organization and address specific unit CRM needs. These two-to-four-hour workshops are generally conducted in smaller groups of 10 to 15 people. Typical workshops cover communication strategies, conflict management, checklist design, and leadership development. These workshops become a permanent part of the organization's CRM curriculum, repeated as necessary.

Phase 4. Facilitated Debriefs

The goal of this phase is to observe teams in action and provide feedback to team members and the organization. Briefing and debriefing sessions also can be conducted in association with simulated activities. Briefings clarify who will be leading the team, prepare the team for the flow of the procedure, delineate expectations, and provide opportunities to discuss potential contingency plans (Healy, Barker, and Madonna 2006). Healthcare team briefings and debriefings take little time to perform, help build shared team mental models, and reduce errors, when performed as indicated in Sidebars 4.2 and 4.3 (Musson and Helmreich 2004, Kern 2001).

Phase 5. CRM Coaching

The purpose of ongoing coaching is to sustain momentum and help teams overcome obstacles. Research in both aviation and healthcare indicates that an organization will revert to old habits if no one reinforces organizational change (Kern 2001). After implementation of CRM training in 1994, the Army realized a 50 percent reduction in accidents. However, without ongoing training and coaching, the accident rate reverted to preintervention rates within five years (Grubb, Morey, and Simon 2001). Individual coaching for key leaders and change agents provides the skill set to nurture desired CRM behaviors and embed change throughout organizations.

Phase 6. Outcomes Assessments

The goal of this phase is to determine the efficacy of the cultural change process using a pretest and posttest model. Results from this phase are used to update and make appropriate changes to the CRM program. The initial program will last 12 to 18 months, depending on organizational size and complexity. However, true cultural change takes longer, requiring ongoing training and feedback, as discussed in Phase 5, above.

Unique Challenges of Applying CRM to Healthcare

Adapting aviation safety programs to healthcare requires an understanding of the differences between the professions. Organizations such as the Federal Aviation Administration (FAA) develop and

Sidebar 4.2: Healthcare Team Briefing Format

- Write out team member names
- Clarify team member roles and responsibilities and state expected outcome
- Obtain consensus on task to be performed
- Promote open communication
    - Encourage team members to ask questions to clear up ambiguities
    - Ask team members to please speak up if uncomfortable with any aspect of a task
- Identify potential problems
    - Brief team regarding contingencies for potential problems
- End with, "Any Questions?"

Sidebar 4.3: Debriefing Format

- Review
    - What went well?
    - Preferences for amendment based on what could have gone better
    - Team's communication processes and outcomes
    - Ability of team to share the same mental model
- Focus on *team*, not individual issues
- End with, "What did we learn to improve individual and team performance next time?"

---

enforce aviation regulations, and the National Transportation Safety Board (NTSB) investigates accidents. Furthermore, in aviation, the Aviation Safety Reporting System (ASRS) reports near misses and errors that impact safety. Widespread use of medical guidelines and acceptance of a process for reporting all medical errors that is not subject to legal discovery have not yet occurred (Gallagher and Levinson 2005).

Examples of teamwork failure in medical settings include failures to brief team of plans for operation, speak out regarding potential work overload or patient concerns, discuss alternatives and advocate a course of action, establish leadership and resolve conflicts, debrief actions after performing procedures, and provide adequate team training and supervision for residents and other new healthcare professionals (Helmreich and Merritt 1998). Barriers to implementing healthcare CRM training include

- a blaming culture,
- lack of sustained leadership,
- limited physician engagement, and
- inadequate funding of safety initiatives.

The tradeoffs between safety and productivity create a dynamic tension in a profession that celebrates autonomy. Healthcare professionals face difficult transitions changing their status from craftsmen to people who value safety and interchangeability (Amalberti et al. 2005).

CONCLUSION

Physicians, nurses, and administrators ultimately need to function as leaders of high-performance teams (Healy, Barker, and Madonna 2006). By adopting teamwork principles embodied in CRM programs, healthcare workers can learn to break error chains and achieve improved safety levels, similar to the transition that occurred in the airline industry over the last two decades, in which the risk of airline fatality decreased over 30 percent (Leape 1999). A commercial airline pilot exclaimed, "I can fly with anyone," by using a common vocabulary, checklist, and briefing and debriefing techniques. The need for improved collaboration and higher reliability in healthcare is evident. Perhaps through more widespread use of the techniques outlined in this chapter and by commencing CRM training early in training, physicians, nurses, administrators, and other healthcare professionals can make the same claim as the pilot without appearing arrogant (Musson and Helmreich 2004).

KEY CONCEPTS

- Crew Resource Management demonstrates potential for improving outcomes by facilitating collaboration and building a culture that emphasizes safety.
- Effective communication pays dividends in many areas of healthcare by
  - improving outcomes and cutting expenses associated with preventable medical errors, and
  - facilitating recruitment, retention, and competitive positioning.

REFERENCES

AHRQ. 2005. "Safety Climate Survey." [Online publication; retrieved 3/25/05] http://www.ihi.org/NR/rdonlyres/145C099B-5FB4-46EA-8CFD-D08D3CE9082C/1704/SafetyClimateSurvey1.pdf

Amalberti, R., Y. Auroy, D.M. Berwick, and P. Barach. 2005. "Five System Barriers to Achieving Ultrasafe Health Care." *Annals of Internal Medicine* 142 (9): 756–64.

Berwick D.M., and L.L. Leape. 1999. "Reducing Error in Medicine." *British Medical Journal* 319 (7203): 136–37.

Edmondson, A.C., R. Bohmer, and G.P. Pisano. 2001. "Speeding Up Team Learning." *Havard Business Review* 79(10): 125–32.

Gallagher, T.H., and W. Levinson. 2005. "Disclosing Harmful Medical Errors to Patients: A Time for Professional Action. *Archives of Internal Medicine* 165 (16): 1819–24.

Grogan, E.L., R.A. Stiles, D.J. France, T. Speroff, J.A. Morris, B. Nixon, F.A. Gaffney, R. Seddon, and C.W. Pinson. 2004. "The Impact of Aviator-Based

Teamwork Training on the Attitudes of Healthcare Professionals. *Journal of the American College of Surgeons* 199 (6): 843–48.

Grubb, G., J. Morey, and R. Simon. 2001. "Sustaining and Advancing Performance Improvements Achieved by Crew Resource Management Training." *Proceedings of the Eleventh International Symposium on Aviation Psychology*, edited by M.S. Patankar. St. Louis, MO: Parks College of Engineering and Aviation, Saint Louis University.

Healy, G.B., J. Barker, and G. Madonna. 2006. "Error Reduction Through Team Leadership: Applying Aviation's Team Model in the OR." *Bulletin of the American College of Surgeons* 91 (2): 10–15.

Helmreich, R.L., and A.S. Merritt. 1998. *Culture at Work in Aviation and Medicine: National, Organizational, and Professional Influences.* Aldershot, UK: Ashgate.

Kern, T. 2001. *Culture, Environment, & CRM.* New York: McGraw-Hill.

Kohn, L., J. Corrigan, and M. Donaldson (eds.). 2000. *To Err Is Human: Building a Safer Health System.* Committee on Quality of Healthcare in America, Institute of Medicine. Washington, D.C.: National Academies Press.

Leape, L.L. 1999. "Aviation Safety: Use the Right Numbers." [Online article; retrieved 11/12/05.] http://bmj.bmjjournals.com/cgi/eletters/319/7203/136.

Musson, D.M., and R.L. Helmreich. 2004. "Team Training and Resource Management in Healthcare: Current Issues and Future Directions." *Harvard Health Policy Review* 5 (1): 25–35.

Reason, J. 2000. "Human Error: Models and Management. *British Medical Journal.* 320 (7237): 768–70.

CHAPTER 5

Socioeconomic Issues Affecting Healthcare Collaboration

Kenneth H. Cohn, C. Duane Dauner, and Thomas R. Allyn

> Poorly aligned incentives are tearing healthcare professionals apart. The only low-hanging fruit left on the vine is collaboration based on relationships that are grounded in dialogue, transparency, trust, and the pursuit of mutually compatible, patient-centered goals.
>
> —C. Duane Dauner

INTRODUCTION

It is both a curse and a blessing to live in times of rapid change. The curse involves dealing with rapid technological and marketplace change, which makes it necessary but difficult to plan for an uncertain future. As physician and facility reimbursement stagnates or declines, mounting pressures such as regulation; the threat of litigation; consumer pressures; and aging patient, physician, and nursing demographics threaten healthcare professionals' ability to provide high-quality, cost-effective, mission-based services to their communities.

Caught up in the daily siege, with little or no time to reflect, healthcare professionals may find it difficult (to paraphrase an old joke) to find the pony near the manure. Christensen and Stephenson (2005) wrote that the perception of failure and crisis shifts organizations away from consensus and toward command-and-control leadership, which rarely succeeds in the long-term. Healthcare professionals must work smarter by collaborating to create a system that optimizes efficiency and effectiveness for *all* parties.

The blessing of living in an era of disruptive change may lie in the opportunity to rethink the way we care for patients and respond more rapidly to patients' and families' changing wants and needs. In so doing, we can achieve competitive differentiation, increase market share, improve patient care, and boost patient, employee, and physician retention. The purpose of this chapter is to discuss several current issues in healthcare—poorly aligned incentives, uninsured and underinsured patients, governmental underpayment, workforce shortages, and excessive administrative costs affecting healthcare collaboration—and explore ways that healthcare professionals can improve care and their practice environment by working more interdependently. The following case illustrates the difficulty and the importance of bringing together payers, physicians, hospital executives, insurers, patients, and politicians to have a facilitated discussion of healthcare problems and possible reforms.

CASE PRESENTATION

The Pittsburgh Regional Healthcare Initiative (PRHI 2005) began in 1997 when former Treasury Secretary Paul O'Neill and Jewish Healthcare Foundation President Karen Wolk Feinstein assembled a consortium of over 40 hospitals, four major insurers, dozens of small and large businesses, and corporate and civic leaders to improve healthcare for patients and ameliorate the financial picture for those who pay for healthcare. Ms. Feinstein announced: "The issue at the time was the cost of healthcare. We wanted to draw attention to the fact that we thought regions didn't have to wait for a national solution to the increasing costs of healthcare but could fashion a solution locally within their own region" (Savary and Crawford-Mason 2006).

Two factors differentiated PRHI from other models:

1. *Regional collaboration:* PRHI facilitates professionally safe neutral working groups where leaders can share information on improvements rapidly throughout the region across competitive lines. These groups, which form and disband freely according to interest and participation, currently include cardiac surgery, critical care, emergency medicine, chronic conditions, infection control, and long-term care.

2. *Perfecting Patient Care*™: PRHI, as a community resource, teaches this healthcare adaptation of the Toyota Production System (TPS) to personnel from the executive suite to the front line, demonstrating methods for standardizing work and reducing errors and waste. Beginning in 2006, PRHI's founding organization, the Jewish Healthcare Foundation of Pittsburgh, is awarding grants to physicians in select specialty areas who agree to apply Perfecting Patient Care principles to their work and measure their results.

Results to date include:

• A 63-percent regionwide reduction in bloodstream infections associated with the use of intravenous catheters; these infections carry an approximate 50-percent mortality and $30,000 cost to treat. Several individual hospital units in the region have approached zero central line–associated bloodstream infections, and have sustained that rate for over two years.

• Decreased regional readmissions following coronary artery bypass surgery; pooled regional data revealed a 17-percent readmission rate prior to intervention, largely due to postoperative infection; the 4.7-percent decrease in readmission rate is estimated to have saved the region $1.7 million (PRHI 2005).

CASE ANALYSIS

PRHI began with the agreement that the core of every medical endeavor must be the patient's safety and well being, with the provision of the best care every time. Based on this premise, PRHI established regional goals that included

- zero medication errors; and
- zero nosocomial (healthcare-acquired) infections; and
- perfect clinical outcomes, as measured by complications and readmissions, in coronary artery bypass surgery and chronic conditions, such as depression and diabetes.

Many healthcare professionals found the concept of perfection insulting and unrealistic, fearing that it would raise expectations and increase clinicians' risk of lawsuits. It took years for clinicians to view the goal from the patient's perspective and ask, "How many errors are allowable?" and "Who would volunteer for a lottery to be harmed or have harm inflicted on family members?" Gradually, the questions moved from accusatory, "Why don't *you* ...?," to a systems-based reflection, "What if *we* ... ," which formed the basis of the Perfecting Patient Care method that sought to improve patient care one encounter at a time (Grunden 2005).

To watch the work at the Pittsburgh VA Healthcare System, where Perfecting Patient Care began, was to see actual system improvements implemented from the ground up rather than by executive decree. Not only did one unit report an 85-percent reduction in the incidence of methicillin-resistant staphylococcus aureus infection, but improvements "leaked out" to other areas in the three-hospital system, where medication delivery improved to a 99-percent on-time rate, for example.

As improvements surfaced, the prevailing mindset changed from, "We can't afford improved quality without higher spending" to "Quality costs less—a lot less!" People learned of the close interrelationships in the processes of care and began to understand how improved collaboration based on empirical change and observation could improve not only the quality of clinical care but also worker safety and satisfaction, efficiency, revenues, and expenses.

Clearly, it takes time for clinical champions to emerge and to learn to ask the right questions. Some groups, like orthopedics, have disbanded, but others like the PRHI cardiac registry, have become powerful forces, uniting competing specialists to pool data in a blinded fashion to answer questions that single hospitals lack the volume to answer. The model Northern New England Cardiovascular Disease Study Group (2005) has logged data on over 150,000 consecutive procedures since its founding in 1987.

Currently, PRHI is aligning its effort according to the following principles:

- Applying Perfecting Patient Care to transform acute, long-term, and community care settings
- Demonstrating savings that can accrue with providing what the patient needs without error or waste
- Building support among medical specialties to apply lessons from demonstration projects to specialist groups and provider associations
- Transforming reporting, reimbursement, and regulatory systems to focus on activities that make the biggest differences in improving quality, safety, and efficiency

COMPLEX RESPONSIVE PROCESSES

Understanding complexity in healthcare may help health professionals make sense of their experience and work more productively together (Cohn 2005). Stacey (2003) proposed the term "complex responsive processes" to describe the way in which communication and power relationships emerge in organizations over time. He felt that formal and informal conversations are important in helping individuals and organizations deal with complexity. This principle underlies the success of the structured dialogue process described in Chapter 1 and creative abrasion in Chapter 2, where scheduled meetings among physicians and hospital leaders became forums for formal and informal conversations that improved communication and hospital processes.

Furthermore, Stacey (2003) wrote that learning inevitably leads to anxiety, because challenges to a person's identity are threatening. People cannot know in advance what patterns of identity they are moving into, which may feel like incompetence and failure. In a social order that prizes knowledge and competence and punishes failure, people can feel ashamed about not knowing. Therefore, the challenge facing organizations in times of rapid change is how to create a safe environment for learning (Stacey 1996). For example, one community hospital hosts interdisciplinary conferences called MLEs, or major learning events, because it found that healthcare professionals are more open to discussing improvement opportunities when they feel that they are in a safe environment for learning.

Interdisciplinary conferences in which all stakeholders are present are key to sustainable healthcare reform (Leape and Berwick 2005). Acknowledging the need for conversations characterized by inquiry rather than advocacy is a prerequisite for sensible action to improve clinical outcomes and maintain economic competitiveness (Garvin and Roberto 2001).

We have both an opportunity and a responsibility to move from disaggregated silos to collaboration based on mutual respect, dialogue, transparency, and win-win negotiation. Local successes can lead to progressive improvement and eventually to enlightened public policy, as described in the case presentation.

Disaggregation

"Disaggregation" is a state in which people who need to work interdependently fail to do so because of lack of time, lack of understanding of the context in which they operate, or unwillingness to recognize that their assumptions are not valid. Disaggregation flourishes in an environment of poorly aligned incentives, in which people who make an extra effort to improve patient care are not uniformly recognized or rewarded (Porter and Teisberg 2004); disaggregation affects every aspect of the provision of healthcare, as described below. Physicians lose time, hospitals lose money, and patients can suffer adverse outcomes (Kohn, Corrigan, and Donaldson 2000; Leape and Berwick 1999).

Physician Perspectives: A Different Approach to Gainsharing

Although poorly aligned incentives may have been around for decades, their effects seem more noticeable in the current environment. A cardiac surgeon quipped, "As the portions get smaller, the table manners deteriorate," to express his frustration with being squeezed between stagnant or declining reimbursement and rising expenses, and with feeling that his time and service were less valued than in the past. The deteriorating economic situation leaves healthcare professionals feeling isolated and detached from the implications of their actions and inactions, especially if the only solution to maintaining their incomes involves working harder to see and treat more patients.

Hospitals throughout the United States lose revenue when expenses exceed reimbursement for Medicare inpatients; these losses increase when Medicare patients are allowed to stay over a weekend until their regular physician discharges them. Moreover, keeping patients in the hospital longer than necessary increases the risk of hospital-acquired infections and adverse drug reactions (Leape and Berwick 2005).

Healthcare professionals need to continue to work to change current payment policies and systems of care. If discharge planners at hospitals and receiving facilities such as rehabilitation centers and nursing homes were available to expedite discharges on weekends and holidays, perhaps weekend and holiday discharges might become more routine. Healthcare professionals generally welcome changes that make more effective use of their time if framed in a manner that shows the benefits to them and their patients.

Gainsharing offers an incentive to alter clinical decision making. Although aspects of gainsharing that transfer income to physicians are in their legal infancy (Becker 2005), to date, the authors are not aware of laws that prevent hospital executives from showing practicing physicians what revenue the hospital loses and what funds, for example, could be reinvested in clinical capital budget projects if lengths of stay are reduced. This virtual gainsharing limits both the possibility of audits from the Office of the Inspector General and toxic incentives, in which clinicians come to expect annual stipends for patient care improvement efforts (Berwick 1995).

Administrative Costs: Departmental Silos, Costs of Contracting, and Regulations

Hospitals are complex organizations in which many people interact, and in the process of that interaction change the context for other participants (Cohn 2005). Organizational charts reflect a more idealized notion of communication than occurs in complex organizations, where effective management requires dotted-line collaboration within areas of influence more than administrative control. Yet, departmental silos, especially in the budgeting process, make collaboration more of a nicety than a necessity (Lambert 2004).

Contracting has not optimized payer-provider collaboration. Despite calls for cost containment, the current system has the opposite effect. The additional costs of rules that do not add value to patient care extend throughout the clinical and administrative sides of the hospital. For example, Kahn et al. (2005) estimated that 20 to 22 percent of the spending on physician and hospital services in California that is paid through private insurance is used for billing and insurance-related functions.

The estimated $470 billion spent per year on administrative expenses subtracts funds that could be used to improve access and care (Woolhandler and Himmelstein 1997). Lewis (2001) wrote that we could provide care for our nation's uninsured for approximately $190 billion annually; by decreasing time to detection and treatment, this provision might also decrease overall healthcare costs. Similarly, if startup costs for electronic medical records average $15 to 20 million per hospital (Carpenter 2002), computerized medical records might be implemented in U.S. hospitals for approximately $100 billion. If the current system grows more expensive, it will become unsustainable and may limit our options for reform. Already, both industry and labor complain that rising healthcare expenses limit U.S. global competitiveness (Klepper and Salber 2005).

Additional Perspectives: Governmental Mandates, Education, and Politics

Other areas where collaboration could improve current problems include the following.

Medicaid

A combination of federal and state regulations makes more work for caregivers and frequently drives a wedge between healthcare professionals caught between the demands of their practices and a mandate to provide emergency care (Fong 2005).

On-call issues involving care for the uninsured and the underinsured result in conflicts of ED physicians against specialists and older members of physician groups against younger members and have resulted in hospitals paying physicians to obtain 24/7 coverage, a service that once was considered an obligation in return for membership on the medical staff. California hospitals paid physicians over $600 million to serve as members of on-call panels in 2005, according to the California Healthcare Association (2005).

Assistance for Small Businesses

Outsourcing healthcare to a larger organization that pools risk needs further encouragement; the purpose of insurance is to gain predictability by spreading losses over large numbers of insured workers (Feldstein 2005). Such a system might decrease the number of uninsured or underinsured workers and improve overall workers' wellness through timely management of conditions such as hypertension and diabetes (Klepper and Salber 2005, Lee and Zapert 2005).

Increased Incentives for Employers to Augment Wellness Programs

Researchers are beginning to recognize the benefits of chronic disease management in patients with heart conditions and asthma; why are similar connections not sought for obesity, to limit the number of patients needing future treatment for diabetes, joint destruction, high blood pressure, and kidney failure (Olshansky et al. 2005)?

Education

Future healthcare consumers are inadequately taught how to choose nutritious foods, evaluate health plans, judge quality, and protect their own and their relatives' healthcare safety (Wilson and Sheikh 2002, Lee and Zapert 2005).

Insurers

Efforts to encourage physicians and hospital executives to work more interdependently with insurers could improve systems of care and decrease variation in healthcare utilization (Wennberg et al. 2005).

Payers' report cards on physicians and hospital executives also exacerbate disaggregation by focusing on multiple standards, rather than establishing a uniform rating system that is standard across all payers (Elder and Dovey 2002, Khuri 2005)

Elected Officials

Because of the reaction to comprehensive healthcare reform in 1994 and the difficulty of holding individual members account-able for spending decisions, elected officials have chosen to tin-ker at the edges with self-serving legislation (Fuchs and Emanuel 2005). For example, Medicare drug coverage increases expenses without providing comparable operational savings or promoting heightened collaboration and shortens the time until our non-system of healthcare becomes bankrupt.

Workforce Shortages

The supply of caregivers and allied healthcare professionals is not keeping pace with the demand for hospital care. For example, as of December 2004, hospitals estimated the number of vacant posi-tions for registered nurses was 109,000, approximately 8 percent of all part-time and full-time nursing positions (Steinberg 2006). An increase in the supply of nurses is important to the ability to meet the demands for care. However, from 1995 to 1999, the num-ber of nursing graduates declined 13.6 percent, and the median age of existing nurses rose to over 43 years (AONE 2001). Only 10 percent of the nursing workforce is under 30. Women, who account for 92.8 percent of registered nurses, are 40 percent less likely to enter the nursing profession now than 20 years ago (Dasso and Wilson 2001). Moreover, the number of registered nurses who are no longer working in nursing has risen 22 percent, from 387,000 in 1992 to 494,000 in 2000 (Jaffe 2001).

Raising wages, decreasing education costs, and upgrading the image of nursing are long-term strategies to correct the nursing shortage; however, the impact of these interventions is unlikely to be felt in time to alleviate the growing shortage. Nor is importing nurses from other countries a viable long-term strategy. Instead, improving surgeon-nurse partnerships by managing disruptive physician behavior (Erickson, Warshaw, and Ditomassi 2002) and redesigning work to enable an aging workforce to be more efficient at providing and documenting care, and using revised patient-care algorithms and hand-held or voice-activated technology appear to be promising solutions (AONE 2001).

CONCLUSION

The present global economic squeeze, poorly aligned incentives that pit groups against each other, and the failure of politicians to undertake systematic healthcare reform inhibit collaboration and add expense to an already overburdened non-system of healthcare. Meetings of all major stakeholders that provide a forum for discussion and sharing rather than blaming can help deal with the complexity in healthcare and improve clinical and financial outcomes.

KEY CONCEPTS

- It is time to bring payers, physicians, hospital executives, insurers, patients, and politicians together to have a facilitated discussion of healthcare problems and necessary reforms.

- Understanding complexity and the need for conversations characterized by inquiry rather than advocacy is a prerequisite for sensible action to improve clinical outcomes and maintain economic competitiveness.
- Effective dialogue and collaboration are no longer niceties but necessities.
- Reforms must address currently unresolved issues in healthcare: poorly aligned incentives, uninsured and underinsured patients, governmental underpayment, excessive administrative costs, and workforce shortages.

REFERENCES

American Organization of Nurse Executives. 2001. "Tricare Strategies to Reverse the New Nursing Shortage: A Policy Statement of the American Association of Critical Care Nurses (AACN), American Nurses Association (ANA), American Organization of Nurse Executives (AONE), and National League for Nursing (NLN)." [Online article; created 1/31/01; retrieved 2/24/06.] http://www.aone.org/news/tricouncil_shortage%20strategies.htm.

Becker, C. 2005. "Device Costs Go Under the Knife." *Modern Healthcare* 35 (8): 6–7,16.

Berwick DM. "The Toxicity of Pay for Performance." *Quality Management in Health Care* 4 (1): 27–33.

California Healthcare Association. 2005. Internal Survey of Members. Unpublished data.

Carpenter, D. 2002. "The Paperless Chase: Hospitals Seek to Cross the Digital Divide with EMRs." *Hospital and Health Networks* 76 (1): 47–48.

Christensen, C., and H. Stephenson. 2005. "The Tools of Cooperation." Harvard Business School Case 9-399-080, rev. February 21, 1–12.

Cohn, K.H. 2005. "Embracing Complexity." *Better Communication for Better Care: Mastering Physician-Administrator Collaboration*, 30–38. Chicago: Health Administration Press.

Dasso, E., and T. Wilson. 2001. "New Model Helps Find Missing Link Between Financial and Clinical Health Management. *Physician Executive* 27 (6): 51–56.

Elder, N.C., and S.M. Dovey. 2002. "Classification of Medical Errors and Preventable Adverse Effects in Primary Care: A Synthesis of the Literature." *Journal of Family Practice* 51 (11): 927–32. Erratum 51 (12): 1079.

Erickson, J.I., A.L. Warshaw, and M. Ditomassi. 2002. "The Health Care Worker Shortage: Suggested Responses from the Surgical Community." *Bulletin of the American College of Surgeons* 86 (6):13–18.

Feldstein, P.J. 2005. *Health Care Economics, 6th ed*, 194. Clifton Park, NY: Thomson Delmar Learning.

Fong, T. 2005. "Assessing Four Decades of Medicare, Medicaid." *Modern Healthcare* 35 (29): 6–7,24,42.

Fuchs, V.R., and E.J. Emanuel. 2005. "Health Care Reform: Why? What? When?" *Health Affairs* 24 (6): 1399–1414.

Garvin, D.A., and M.A. Roberto. 2001. "What You Don't Know About Making Decisions." *Harvard Business Review* 79 (8): 108–15.

Grunden, N. 2005. "The Pittsburgh Regional Healthcare Initiative: Trials and Triumphs of the Early Years Point the Way Toward the Future." Unpublished manuscript.

Jaffe, B.M. 2001. "Where Have All the Nurses Gone?" *Surgical Rounds* 24 (6): 290–91.

Kahn, J.G., R. Kronick, M. Kreger, and D.N. Gans. 2005. "The Cost of Health Insurance Administration in California: Estimates for Insurers, Physicians, and Hospitals." *Health Affairs* 24 (6): 1629–39.

Khuri, S. 2005. "The NSQIP: A New Frontier in Surgery." *Surgery* 138 (5): 837–43.

Klepper, B., and P. Salber. 2005. "The Business Case for Reform." *Modern Healthcare* 35 (41): 22.

Kohn, L., J. Corrigan, and M. Donaldson (eds). 2000. *To Err Is Human: Building a Safer Health System*. Committee on Quality of Healthcare in America, Institute of Medicine. Washington, D.C.: National Academies Press.

Lambert, M. 2004. "Improvement and Innovation in Hospital Operations: A Key to Organizational Health." *Frontiers of Health Services Management* 20 (4): 39–45.

Leape, L.L., and D.M. Berwick. 1999. "Reducing Errors in Medicine." *British Medical Journal*. 319 (7203): 136–37.

Lee, T.H., and K. Zapert. 2005. "Do High-Deductible Plans Threaten Quality of Care?" *New England Journal of Medicine*. 353 (12): 1202–204.

Lewis, F.R. 2001. "Costs, Competence, and Consumerism: Challenges to Medicine in the New Millennium." *Journal of Trauma* 50 (2): 185–94.

Northern New England Cardiovascular Disease Study Group. 2005. [Online material, retrieved 12/23/05.] http://www.nnecdsg.org/about.htm.

Olshansky, S.J., D.J. Passaro, R.C. Hershow, J. Layden, B.A. Carnes, J. Brody, L. Hayflick, R.N. Butler, D.B. Allison, and D.S. Ludwig. "A Potential Decline in Life Expectancy in the United States in the 21st Century." *New England Journal of Medicine* 352 (11): 1138–45.

Pittsburgh Regional Healthcare Initiative (PRHI). 2005. "Background: Executive Summary." [Online article; retrieved 11/28/05.] http://www.prhi.org/ourmodel.cfm

Porter, M.E., and E.O. Teisberg. 2004. "Redefining Competition in Health Care." *Harvard Business Review* 82 (6): 64–76.

Savary, L.M., and C. Crawford-Mason. 2006. *The Nun and the Bureaucrat: How They Found a Simple, Elegant Solution to a Deadly National Healthcare Problem*, 12. Washington, D.C.: CC-M Productions, Inc.

Stacey, R.D. 2003. *Complexity and Group Processes: A Radically Social Understanding of Individuals*, 297–98. New York: Brunner-Routledge.

———. 1996. "Emerging Strategies for a Chaotic Environment." *Long Range Planning* 29 (2): 182–89.

Steinberg, C.R. 2006. "Trends: An Overview of 2004." *AHA Hospital Statistics*, xvii–xix. Chicago: Health Forum, LLC.

Wennberg, J.E., E.S. Fisher, L. Baker, S.M. Sharp, and K.K. Bronner. 2005. "Evaluating the Efficiency of California Providers in Caring for Patients with Chronic Illness." *Health Affairs*. [Online article; retrieved 11/16/05.] http://content.healthaffairs.org/cgi/content/abstract/hlthaff.w5.526v1.

Wilson,T., and A. Sheikh. 2002. "Enhancing Public Safety in Primary Care." *British Medical Journal* 324 (7337): 584–87.

Woolhandler, S., and D.U. Himmelstein. 1997. "Costs of Care and Administration at For-Profit and Other Hospitals." *New England Journal of Medicine* 336 (11): 769–74. Erratum 337 (24): 1783.

CHAPTER 6

Changing the Rules in Health Care Collaboration Using Adaptive Design®

Kenneth H. Cohn, David L. Sundahl, and John Kenagy

> What does it take to get a —ing wheelchair around here?
> Would you want to have your hip replaced in a hospital that can't keep track of its wheelchairs?
> —*A charge nurse at a Midwestern community teaching hospital*

INTRODUCTION

Traditional quality improvement strategies have involved managers designing projects for frontline workers to perform. A problem with top-down approaches is that they promote a passive orientation to the workplace and slow worker responsiveness. The purpose of this chapter is to outline the principles of the Toyota Production System as they apply to healthcare. The applicable principles focus on the needs of frontline workers and the benefits of heightened efficiency, improved collaboration, and decreased waste in improving patient care and employee satisfaction.

What Is the Toyota Production System?

The Toyota Production System (TPS) is a system of nested experiments to improve operations on a continuing basis (Spear 2004). The TPS encompasses four rules:

1. All work is highly specified regarding content, sequence, timing, and outcome: each step is described by what to do, why is it being done, when it should occur, how long it should take, and what is the expected result.
2. Every connection between people must be direct and must have a clear way to send requests and receive responses.
3. The pathway for every product and service must be simple and direct: goods and services flow to a specific person, not the next available person, and any suppliers not connected to path are unnecessary.
4. Any improvement must be made in accord with the scientific method, under a teacher's guidance, at the lowest possible organizational level.

PRINCIPLES OF ADAPTIVE DESIGN®

What is Adaptive Design?

Adaptive Design (AD) is a process designed by a physician (author John Kenagy) who apprenticed himself to Toyota for two years to learn the TPS and adapt it to healthcare. Adaptive Design is a method that focuses on meeting the needs of patients by building flexibility into work processes, helping frontline workers expand their problem-solving skills, and using the scientific method to guide improvement efforts. Quality, safety, and improvement become every worker's responsibility (Spear and Bowen 1999).

Adaptive Design is a method to teach the practices and principles of TPS in healthcare environments in a disciplined, repeatable way, using the following principles:

1. Leaders create responsiveness to new conditions by focusing themselves and others on problem-solving activities at the level closest to patients.
2. Improvements must be made as close in time and place to a problem as possible. Frontline workers solve problems based on real-time observations and experiences without forming new committees.
3. Learning the principles of AD occurs through making improvements rather than by attending classes. Issues with immediate impact are the primary opportunities to teach staff, physicians, and managers the skills of improvement, as discussed in the case presentation below.

CASE PRESENTATION

"What does it take to get a —ing wheelchair around here?" the charge nurse asked. "I've got two patients waiting in the post-anesthesia care unit (PACU) for beds, but unit support can't find a wheelchair to discharge a patient in Room 436, and we're waiting for physical therapy to clear another patient in Room 458. Nothing changes around here. Would *you* want to have your hip replaced in a hospital that can't keep track of its wheelchairs?"

Jan was one of three charge nurses on 4E, a 44-bed medical-surgical nursing unit. Although Jan and the other charge nurses were among the most experienced and clinically knowledgeable nurses, they spent over 80 percent of their time "treating the system," including hunting for wheelchairs and blood pressure cuffs, calling physicians, and juggling the discharge and admission process. Her floor nurses spent on average only one-fifth of their time with patients, approximately one-third of their time documenting and reporting as required by national mandates, and the remainder of their time solving system problems such as searching for equipment and supplies (see Table 6.1; Kenagy, Berwick, and Shore 1999).

Jan and others reported that they often found the unit stalled for lack of a wheelchair. To address the problem, some staff searched in places they knew wheelchairs were likely to be "hiding." Others went to other units and furtively "borrowed" a wheelchair. Regardless of the specific method, capable people figured out how to get a wheelchair. Unfortunately, these approaches meant that the underlying problem was not resolved (Tucker and Edmondson 2003). Finding hidden wheelchairs or stealing them from neighboring units met the immediate need but did not correct the systemic cause of the problem.

In an effort to stop applying temporary band-aids, the hospital decided to implement AD. To create a focus on frontline problem solving—the first principle of teaching AD—Jan's leaders did three things: (1) they helped Jan and her manager allocate time to learning and improving work using AD; (2) they provided Jan with a trained teacher of AD; and (3) leaders came to the unit to learn what Jan (and others) were doing and how they could help. These three investments showed staff and physicians that the organization was serious about improving conditions for patients. Leaders communicated and demonstrated their focus on frontline improvement.

With these investments in learning and improvement in place, Jan could work on the second principle of AD—making improvements as close in time and place to a problem as possible. Jan and her teacher quickly helped the unit support person find a wheelchair tucked away in a supply room on the unit, but they also went beyond superficial problem solving. They observed the unit support person discharge a patient and return the wheelchair to the unit, where she left the wheelchair in the hallway. When the teacher asked Jan, "how does she know where to put that wheelchair?," Jan realized that although locations had been written in large letters on the backs of the wheelchairs, that information was insufficient. A 44-bed unit was a big place.

Under the guidance of her teacher and in consultation with nurses and unit support people, Jan decided that the unit should establish wheelchair parking lots and place instructions on each wheelchair regarding where they should be returned. By observing work as it actually happened and by analyzing a problem while it was fresh, Jan was ready to test a solution to her problem of missing wheelchairs.

Jan was learning by doing. Her teacher used the problem of the missing wheelchair as an opportunity to learn. Specifically, Jan learned *how* to use the tools of observation and problem solving. For instance, Jan learned the importance of observation as she discovered new facts about a problem that she thought she understood completely. She learned that the question about how someone knows where to put a wheelchair was not a trivial matter. In the design and implementation phases of the process, Jan's teacher taught her how to design a solution that was self-diagnostic and improvable. Jan reported that the tools and methods described were not new to her; rather, she experienced a new ability to apply the tools and methods to solve problems on her unit.

Another advantage to learning by doing is that as Jan worked through more problems, her skills improved to the point at which she became a teacher. Over the next several months, Jan trained frontline nurses and aides in her unit using opportunities her staff identified. During that period, the unit made over 100 improvements using AD. The staff and unit manager solved problems that ranged from simple and seemingly unimportant to those that were complex and vital. The improvements included

- providing softer toilet paper for patients with skin integrity problems;
- increasing coordination of discharge for orthopedic patients;

- complying with regulations on the return of unused medications to the pharmacy;
- implementing procedures for moving patients safely;
- safely delivering meals for patients whose immune systems were compromised, as well as for other patients on precautions;
- using pump-compatible IV tubing for surgery patients who required infusions of medication; and
- coordinating safe transfer of patients during unit renovations.

The improvements arose from learning by observing and testing solutions, the third principle of AD.

After a few months of improving the work environment, the proportion of nurses' time employed in solving system problems was cut in half, from 43 percent to 22 percent (Table 6.1). One year later, the unit's patient satisfaction scores were the best in the entire system. Moreover, the nurses' attitudes became more realistic and optimistic. They recognized the remaining problems and the power of AD in solving them. As Jan proudly reported, "We're ready for whatever they throw at us."

CASE ANALYSIS

Jan's experience illustrates the three principles that underlie AD's teaching. First, the organization focused on improving conditions at the level closest to patients by helping staff develop their problem-solving skills. Second, the staff solved problems through direct observation as close in time and place to the actual problem as possible without establishing new committees or task forces. Finally, Jan and her colleagues learned by solving problems that mattered to them and their patients.

The process underlying AD differs from traditional management principles in that management in AD develops and

Table 6.1: Changes in Allocation of Nursing Time Using Adaptive Design

	Baseline	4 Months	14 Months
Solving system problems	43%	22%	11%
Documenting	35%	40%	35%
Caring directly for patients	22%	47%	54%

Source: Kenagy, Berwick, and Shore, 1999.

Table 6.2: Comparison of Traditional Management Principles with the Principles of Adaptive Design

	Traditional Management	*Adaptive Design*
Organizational objective(s)	Pursue financial goals and numerical targets	Provide each patient what they need when they need it
Employees	Perceived as a cost to be managed	Perceived as a valued asset
Management	Obtain data from workplace, identify gaps/opportunities, and push solutions	Develop and challenge a workforce to improve its own performance
Decisions	– Made by managers in meetings – Implemented through management-led initiatives – Designed to be followed, not improved	–Made by those with relevant information (may be managers) –Implemented by frontline staff –Tested and improved over time
Improvement	Driven by leaders and done in committees	Driven by frontline staff, primarily in the course of work

Table 6.3: Comparison of Rules for Change and Improvement

	Traditional Management	*Adaptive Design*
How we approach improvement	Access capital; do big projects	Conserve resources; diversify risk
How we motivate people	Set targets; offer incentives	Connect work to purpose
Why we measure	To make the case	To improve
How we grow	Pilot; roll out quickly; be patient for profitability	Seek immediate value; be patient for growth
What we seek	Top-down "fix"	Frontline "fitness"

challenges its workforce to improve its own performance, with improvement efforts driven by frontline staff, primarily in the course of work (Table 6.2). The rules also differ, with emphasis on frontline fitness rather than top-down improvement efforts (Table 6.3). For AD to succeed, leaders also must undergo training, as discussed below.

LEADERSHIP

The power of leadership is a fundamental element of AD. Regular, brief, face-to-face conversations between leaders and their units provide the direction, protection, and order that the unit needs and allow leaders to oversee projects effectively.

Direction is important because it can prevent a unit from wasting time attempting to design "the perfect plan" to reach its vision rather than acting, learning, and adapting. "Perfect plans" become impractical when workers encounter changed circumstances and unforeseen obstacles. As an example of appropriate direction, a hospital CEO scheduled weekly 30-minute visits that enabled him to reinforce principles and to learn from the unit's experience. Once momentum was established, the CEO made less frequent visits. Ultimately, the CEO found that these visits saved him time and effort. His understanding of and standing with the unit increased rapidly.

Protection is important because learning leads to anxiety when people do not know what will be expected of them in their new knowledge roles. At the same time, in a social order that prizes knowledge and punishes failure, people can feel ashamed not to know. Therefore, a challenge facing organizations in times of rapid change is how to create a safe environment for learning (Stacey 1996). In this example, teachers assigned to units could frame questions by asking, "Why," five times to reveal root causes, rather than by asking accusingly, "Why didn't *you* perform up to expectations?" (Grunden 2005).

Order is important because experimentation cannot be done randomly. Improvements should move with discipline and in concert with the rest of the organization. Leaders create order both explicitly and tacitly. For example, they can establish order explicitly through ground rules, such as, "Do the smallest testable experiment possible," and by teaching. They can establish order tacitly by example and by questioning, as with, "How do we know that this change represents an improvement?"

Leaders must set aside small amounts of time to learn about improvement efforts, teach improvement principles, and re-focus staff. By doing so, they will find themselves in a position where they are once again leading.

RATIONALE FOR ADAPTIVE DESIGN IN HEALTHCARE

Adaptive Design meets the needs of patients and healthcare workers in an environment in which rapid change has disrupted conventional ways of working (Christensen, Bohmer, and Kenagy 2000). Signs of current disruption in the healthcare marketplace include:

- loss of profitable services, especially to small, focused provider organizations such as ambulatory surgical centers and specialty hospitals;
- fragmentation of previously stable services; for example, when cardiologists offer outpatient services like nuclear imaging or when orthopedists offer in-office magnetic resonance imaging (MRI) scans that used to be performed within the hospital;
- increasing emphasis on cost-cutting and operational metrics to solve problems that require informal networks to transcend departmental silos;
- scaling down of business or exiting previously profitable areas because of increased marketplace competition;
- restructuring and merger and acquisition activity to create market power or to take capacity out of the marketplace; and
- decreased physician and employee satisfaction, with decreased morale and employee retention.

Adaptive Design offers local solutions to global problems. It builds on employees' expertise and creativity rather than imposing external best practices (Spear 2004). It merits consideration when people feel frustrated by the pace of change and their limited ability to accommodate or be proactive.

RESULTS OF ADAPTIVE DESIGN IN HEALTHCARE

Examples of successes with AD include:

- The pharmacy department of a 250-bed hospital experienced a $1.9-million increase in net income in less than a year, with a 2.3-percent decrease in volume-adjusted drug costs (VADC); during the same period, 11 other pharmacies in the system experienced an 11-percent increase in VADC.

- A medical-surgical unit saved over $1.2 million in one year, while simultaneously placing in the top quartile for Hospital Standardized Mortality Ratio.
- A large multi-specialty unit decreased registered nurse turnover by 51 percent in one year
- In six months, an operative services department added an additional $800,000 to the hospital's net income by processing cases more efficiently, including decreasing turnaround time.
- A surgical services department improved employee engagement, boosted case volume by 16 percent, and cut overtime by 14 percent; when new perioperative infection protocols were introduced, this unit was found to be in 100 percent compliance.

HOW DOES AN ORGANIZATION DECIDE WHETHER ADAPTIVE DESIGN IS A GOOD FIT?

An organization may be ready for AD if:

- Leaders and staff would like to work together more productively and collaboratively, but are not sure where to begin.
- People are open to exploring new ways of working together.
- Leaders want to integrate strategy with operational effectiveness.
- An organization sees the advantages of creating a shared direction.
- An organization is ready to reflect and make difficult choices about which of its practices to change or eliminate.

CONCLUSION

Adaptive Design is a rigorous method for improving the operations, culture, and finances of an organization. It empowers leaders and staff to improve their work and achieve lasting success.

KEY CONCEPTS

- Sustainable improvement starts with frontline workers reflecting and testing new ways to improve processes that affect patient care.
- Leaders and managers provide direction, protection, and order to create an environment conducive to teaching and learning.
- Rapid, AD-based problem solving by frontline workers, leaders, and managers improves collaboration, alignment, and clinical and financial outcomes.

REFERENCES

Christensen, C.M., R. Bohmer, and J. Kenagy. 2000. "Will Disruptive Innovations Cure Health Care?" *Harvard Business Review* 78 (5): 102–11.

Grunden, N. 2005. "Industrial Techniques Help Reduce Hospital-Acquired Infection." *Biomedical Instrumentation and Technology* 39 (5): 386–90 .

Kenagy, J.W., D.L. Sundahl, and J. Udall. 2004. "Delivering on the Promise: An Adaptive Approach to Information Technology in Healthcare." [Microsoft whitepaper online, retrieved 11/1/05.] http://www.microsoft.com/industry/healthcare/adaptivedesign.mspx

Kenagy, J.W., D.M. Berwick, and M.F. Shore. 1999. "Service Quality in Health Care." *Journal of the American Medical Association* 281 (7): 661–65.

Spear, S.J. 2004. "Learning to Lead at Toyota." *Harvard Business Review* 82 (5): 78–86.

Spear, S.J., and S.K. Bowen. 1999. "Decoding the DNA of the Toyota Production System." *Harvard Business Review* 77 (5): 95–106.

Stacey, R. 1996. "Emerging Strategies for a Chaotic Environment." *Long Range Planning* 29 (2): 182–89.

Tucker, A.L., and A.C. Edmondson. 2003. "Why Hospitals Don't Learn from Failures: Organizational and Psychological Dynamics that Inhibit System Change." *California Management Review* 45: 55–72.

CHAPTER 7

Let's Do Something: A Cutting-Edge Collaboration Strategy

Kenneth H. Cohn, Sharon Cannon, and Carol Boswell

Do not go where the path may lead. Go instead where there is no path, and leave a trail.

—*Ralph Waldo Emerson*

INTRODUCTION

Nurses are vital contributors to the strategic partnerships necessary to solve current healthcare problems (Boswell and Cannon 2005). No one group has the knowledge, time, or energy to provide and monitor all aspects of patient care. The Institute of Medicine publication *Keeping Patients Safe* (2004) demonstrated decreases in length of stay, more favorable perception of teamwork, and improved understanding of the patient care plan resulting from interdisciplinary team rounds. It concluded, "Clearly, interpersonal communication, regard for others, a strong focus on patient safety goals, and constant reassessment of the environment are important aspects of the relationship between team performance and care delivery outcomes."

The purpose of this chapter is to showcase the progress made by leveraging strategic collaboration to improve clinical outcomes.

Employing hospital administrators, nurse educators, and community leaders in innovative approaches provides solutions that are applicable to multiple healthcare settings.

CASE PRESENTATION

The "Let's Do Something" (LDS) approach was created from a nurse's self-challenge and grew to encompass 19 organizations. It began in 2001 when three nurses met to discuss nursing shortages in their communities. They identified several clinical opportunities. They networked with hospitals, school districts, community colleges, and the chambers of commerce in two neighboring communities to establish a Health Careers Consortium (HCC). The team made a recruitment video to show at high school job fairs and a coloring book for local grade-school children to encourage them to consider healthcare careers. Each of the HCC meetings included an agenda item termed "community update." During these updates, hospital personnel identified problem areas and needs and asked for ideas or suggestions for help. In many instances, community members also asked the nurse educators for input into community program development.

Within the area, community college nursing programs had reduced their operating room content, which was viewed as a specialty. Hospital executives identified a critical need for OR nurses and went back to their supporting organizations with a shared vision to unite community leaders, develop innovative strategies, and stimulate OR nurse recruitment and retention. Staff nurses at three hospitals participated in a pilot program that used four acute care facilities within a 150 mile radius for training. Each hospital identified staff nurses to train to be OR circulators. The nurses retained their salaries while attending the course. Each participant received textbooks for the course from a grant. Participants learned the circulator role in several different venues to optimize training. All 13 of the participants completed the course work and returned to work as OR circulating nurses at their facilities.

From this collaboration, another opportunity arose related to magnet status for acute care facilities. This project endeavored to address the criteria for seeking magnet status by the major acute care agencies within the community. One area of concern has been the use and conduct of research by nursing personnel. A six-week introductory research course was provided to the nursing staff to reflect the importance of evidence-based practice. From this course, a research project was proposed to identify the understanding concerning evidence-based practice and the use of research by staff nurses.

Obtaining magnet status for hospitals is a means to recruit and retain qualified nursing personnel. The direct involvement of nursing personnel in self-government is a key aspect. By participating in courses on research, administrative nursing personnel were engaged in direct discussion concerning evidence-based nursing practice. Research opportunities that benefit the healthcare team and result in improved patient outcomes are a direct outcome of this program. Hospital executives profit from the active engagement of the nursing staff in providing quality healthcare and improving patient outcomes.

CASE ANALYSIS

Mason (2005) asserted that people are only as powerful as they believe themselves to be. LDS is based on the mutually reinforcing principles of vision, leadership, and networking that facilitate collaboration.

Vision

A vision is a clear and compelling picture of the future that people care about bringing to reality. A vision builds community by bonding people of diverse races, religions, ages, and lifestyles in a shared purpose (Atchison 2006). Vision inspires people to believe that they can accomplish something worthwhile and serves as an anchor in difficult times. A vision helps organizations differentiate their service from competitors' and can aid in recruiting and retention (Hoover 2001).

Vision allows for members of a group to come together with a common mission for a project. By making the time and energy to establish shared expectations, the group increases its chances of success. When everyone is involved in the establishment of a shared vision, each member takes ownership of the work (Schaefer 2004).

LDS flourished when three nurses developed a shared vision with a consortium of community leaders to use innovative approaches in hospitals and schools to address critical nursing shortages. The vision for one issue propelled other people into action on additional issues focused on community healthcare needs. Competition among hospitals for market share occurs, but improving care for the community remains at the forefront for the consortium.

A successful vision must be (Hoover 2001)

1. clear, without jargon or corporate doublespeak;
2. consistent, reflecting knowledge of people, the industry, and national and local trends;
3. unique, satisfying unmet needs, executed with passion and intensity; and
4. service-oriented, maintaining focus on what is best for patients and families.

These four characteristics underscore the importance of leadership.

Leadership

After establishing a shared vision, leaders must turn vision into reality. Leadership is the art of instilling in people the desire to strive together to create a better future (Souba 2000). Leaders listen, observe, provide direction and meaning, generate and sustain trust, convey hope, and obtain results through their influence on other employees, according to Warren Bennis (Kurtzman 1997). According to Kerfoot (2001), the challenge is to energize people to push themselves beyond what they thought they could do.

Resonant Leadership

Goleman and colleagues (2002) defined resonant leaders as people who are attuned to their employees' feelings and move them in a positive direction. Connecting with workers at an emotional level makes work more meaningful and facilitates retention. Four leadership styles create resonance that boosts performance (Goleman, Boyatzis, and McKee 2002):

1. **Visionary** leaders articulate where a group is going, but not how it gets there, inspiring employees to innovate, experiment, and take prudent risks. Empathy, the ability to sense what employees feel and to understand their perspectives, allows visionary leaders to inspire others to set stretch goals and achieve breakthrough results. As John Kenneth Galbraith noted, great leaders had the ability to confront unequivocally the major anxiety of their people in their time (Galbraith 1979).
2. **Coaching** leaders help people identify their unique strengths to achieve their personal and career aspirations.
3. **Affiliative** leaders promote harmony and friendly interactions to build high-performance teams.
4. **Democratic** leaders rely on teamwork, collaboration, and conflict management, using listening skills and empathy to build consensus through participation.

However, two leadership styles diminish resonance (Goleman, Boyatzis, and McKee 2002):

1. **Pacesetting** leaders hold employees to high personal standards by setting an example; when overused, pacesetting can erode morale and cause employees to feel that leaders are out of touch.
2. **Commanding** leaders demand compliance without explaining their rationale; this leadership style may work in emergencies, but its overuse may erode workers' self-esteem and lead to apathy and decreased employee retention. This approach, which physicians-in-training observe frequently, often results in a win-lose approach to managing conflict, rather than a more collaborative approach (Cohn and Peetz 2003).

The most effective leaders use a combination of styles in a transparent, genuine manner (Goffee and Jones 2000):

- Exposing their vulnerability selectively, revealing their approachability and humanity
- Using intuition to gauge the appropriate timing for their proposed course of action
- Revealing their differences to capitalize on what is unique about themselves and their organizations

Transparency

Tobias (2003) used the phrase, "Get the moose on the table," to signal the need to speak openly and transparently about important issues when he was CEO at Eli Lilly. The real challenge for leaders is not communicating, but integrating what they say and write with how they behave. He wrote that having capabilities is necessary but not sufficient. Successful leaders seize opportunities for growth and development, opening the door to more opportunities. He described the need to embrace ambiguity and to recognize that adaptation to change can provide competitive advantage: "Change is a lot like fire.

Manage it, turn it to your advantage, and you will bask in the warmth of its glow; ignore it or manage it poorly, and one thing is certain—you will get burned."

Effective Executives

Drucker (2004) wrote that effective executives varied widely in their personalities, attitudes, values, strengths, and weaknesses, but all followed the same practices:

- They asked, "What needs to be done and what is right for the enterprise?"
- They developed comprehensive action plans.
- They took responsibility for decisions and for communicating.
- They were focused on opportunities rather than problems.
- They ran productive meetings.
- They listened first and spoke last.
- They thought and said "we" rather than "I."

The three nurse leaders employed various leadership styles to accomplish their HCC goals. Their flexibility facilitated collaboration.

Networking

The third component of LDS is networking, where people draw on each other's strengths. Networking is essential for successful completion of group endeavors (Boswell and Cannon 2005).

Bennis (Kurtzman 1997) described the leader's function to find a link between organizations and the outside world: "Leaders are rarely the brightest people in the group. Rather, they have extraordinary taste, which makes them more curators than creators. They are appreciators of talent and nurturers of talent and they have the ability to recognize valuable ideas." Buonocore (2004) wrote that effective leaders know how to surround themselves with the right people as resources. Networking enables leaders to leverage ideas, capital, and expertise to build teams and improve patient care (Boswell and Cannon 2005).

Cross, Liedtka, and Weiss (2005) wrote that an organization is greater than the sum of its parts when business units find a way to harvest innovations resulting from strategic collaboration. Haphazard collaboration can sap people's time and energy and can bog down entire organizations. Informal networks of people with different expertise can help organizations recognize opportunities and challenges and coordinate appropriate responses. Three types of networks added value in the organizations Cross and his colleagues studied:

1. **Custom networks** exist in settings where problems and solutions are ambiguous; they deliver value by quickly framing and solving a problem, often in an innovative way. An example in healthcare might be patient flow issues that involve a variety of departments.
2. **Modular networks** thrive in settings where components of a problem and solution require knowledge and expertise; they deliver value by delivering unique responses, depending on the expertise required. Healthcare examples include surgical teams and regional centers of excellence.
3. **Routine networks** occur in standardized work environments; they deliver value by executing effective and efficient responses to a set of established problems via reliable coordination of relevant expertise. Healthcare examples include information technology call centers and operating room turnaround teams.

Large teams are not essential. LDS began with small groups that used leadership, vision, and networking to surmount obstacles. The key is to involve people who derive pleasure from working with a diverse group united by a common vision. As members develop individual abilities, they become more willing to tackle additional challenges. The enjoyment of collaborating with colleagues from a variety of backgrounds allows everyone to benefit from expanding horizons.

Collaborative Advantage

Kanter (1994) wrote that organizations derive competitive advantage from being able to collaborate effectively. She described the "eight I's that create successful We's," noting that only relationships with full commitment endure long enough to create value for all partners:

1. *Individual excellence:* All parties are strong and have something of value to contribute; they enter into partnering relationships to pursue future opportunities, not to mask weaknesses.
2. *Importance:* All parties want the relationship to work because it fits major strategic objectives.
3. *Interdependence:* All parties need each other because they have complementary assets and skills; neither can accomplish alone what all can do together.
4. *Information:* Partners share what they need to make their relationship work, including goals, objectives, technical data, and knowledge of conflicts, trouble spots, and changing situations.
5. *Investment:* All parties show tangible signs of long-term commitment by devoting resources to their relationship.
6. *Integration:* Partners become teachers and learners; they develop linkages and shared ways of operating at multiple levels of their organizations to work together smoothly.

7. *Institutionalization:* The parties give their relationship a formal status, with clear responsibilities and decision rights that extend beyond the leaders who formed the alliance and thus cannot dissolve on a whim.
8. *Integrity:* Partners behave in honorable ways that justify and enhance transparency and trust.

The LDS Health Careers Consortium exhibited Kanter's emphasis on "we." The group remains a vibrant, viable organization because members transcended individual ego issues to work toward improving healthcare for their communities. Drivers of success included focus, leverage, willingness to take prudent risks, and personal accountability. The success of the group in achieving its goals is reflected in continuing applications for membership from other community organizations.

The Challenge of Complexity

Complexity science studies dynamic interactions in living systems and organizations. One principle from complexity science that is relevant to LDS is non-linearity, in which small efforts can result in large changes (Zimmerman, Lindberg, and Plsek 1998). A fundamental principle for achieving success in complex environments is that in situations characterized by disagreement and uncertainty, the most important thing that we can do is to learn by incorporating the following (Cohn 2005):

1. Encouraging brainstorming and innovative thinking
2. Rewarding intuition and muddling through
3. Striving for effectiveness over efficiency
4. Synthesizing conflicting ideas with an iterative approach:
    • Act, learn, adapt
    • Not expecting to get things right initially

5. Celebrating learning rather than blaming
6. Looking for improved outcomes rather than ideal solutions

CONCLUSION

As healthcare professionals cope with reimbursement and expense challenges, heightened consumerism, and powerful regulatory constraints, vision, leadership, and networking consistently come into play. Each characteristic builds on the previous feature while fueling the development of the next attribute. Energy, persistence, and the celebration of successes sustain the vision.

In difficult times, when resources are tight and people must achieve more with less, LDS allows people to transcend limitations and improve patient care. The approach builds on field-tested principles and conditions that are present in every hospital throughout the country. Where a vision, formal and informal leaders, networks, and prudent risk-takers exist, LDS can provide a framework that allows healthcare professionals to leverage their talents and resources to improve care for their communities.

KEY CONCEPTS

- Let's Do Something uses vision, leadership, and networking to achieve breakthrough results in patient care.
- Success in one area expands the network and facilitates progress in additional areas.
- Drivers of success include:
  - Focus
  - Leverage
  - Willingness to take prudent risks
  - Personal accountability

REFERENCES

Atchison, T.A. 2006. *Leadership's Deeper Dimensions: Building Blocks to Superior Performance*. Chicago: Health Administration Press.

Boswell, C., and S. Cannon. 2005. "New Horizons for Collaborative Partnerships." *Online Journal of Issues in Nursing*. [Online article; created 1/31/05; retrieved 3/29/05.] www.nursingworld.org/ojin/topic26/tpc26_2.htm.

Buonocore, D. 2004. "Leadership in Action: Creating a Change in Practice." *AACN Clinical Issues* 15 (2): 170–81.

Cohn, K.H. 2005. *Better Communication for Better Care: Mastering Physician-Administrator Collaboration*, 30–38. Chicago: Health Administration Press.

Cohn, K.H., and M.E. Peetz. 2003. "Surgeon Frustration: Contemporary Problems, Practical Solutions." *Contemporary Surgery* 59 (2): 76–85.

Cross, R., J. Liedtka, and L. Weiss. 2005. "A Practical Guide to Social Networks." *Harvard Business Review* 83 (3): 124–32.

Drucker, P.F. 2004. "What Makes an Effective Executive?" *Harvard Business Review* 82 (6): 58–63.

Galbraith, J.K. 1979. *The Age of Uncertainty*. Boston: Houghton Mifflin.

Goffee, R., and G. Jones. 2000. "Why Should Anyone Be Led by You?" *Harvard Business Review* 78 (5): 63–70.

Goleman, D., R. Boyatzis, and A. McKee. 2002. *Primal Leadership: Realizing the Power of Emotional Intelligence*. Boston: Harvard Business School Press.

Hoover, G. 2001. *Hoover's Vision: Original Thinking for Business Success*. Independence, KY: Texere.

Institute of Medicine (IOM). 2004. *Keeping Patients Safe: Transforming the Work Environment of Nurses*, 361–63. Washington, DC: National Academies Press.

Kanter, R.M. 1994. "Collaborative Advantage: Successful Partnerships Manage the Relationship, Not Just the Deal." *Harvard Business Review* 72 (4): 96–108.

Kerfoot, K. 2001. "The Art of Raising the Bar. *Dermatology Nursing* 13 (4): 301–302. [Online article; retrieved 11/2/04.] http://gateway.ut.ovid.com/gy1/ovidweb.cgi.

Kurtzman, J. 1997. "An Interview with Warren Bennis." *Strategy & Business* (8): 86–94.

Mason, D.J. 2005. "The Sage Within." *American Journal of Nursing* 105 (5): 11.

Schaefer, K.M. 2004., "Using Business Literature to Illustrate the Power of the Team." *Nurse Educator* 29 (5): 217–19. [Online article; retrieved 11/3/04.] http://gateway.ut.ovid.com/gw1/ovidweb.cgi.

Souba, W.W. 2000. "Editorial: The Core of Leadership." *Journal of Thoracic and Cardiovascular Surgery* 119 (3): 414–19.

Tobias, R., with T. Tobias. 2003. *Put the Moose on the Table.* Bloomington, IN: Indiana University Press.

Zimmerman, B., C. Lindberg, and P. Plsek. 1998. "Edgeware: Insights from Complexity Science for Health Care Leaders." Irving, TX: VHA Inc.

CHAPTER 8

Using Evidence-Based Design to Improve Collaboration, Clinical Outcomes, and Financial Performance

Kenneth H. Cohn and Jain Malkin

This is a once-in-a-lifetime opportunity to get it right. The new hospital can improve care for our community, build our brand, and provide a better place to work for our employees.

—Midwestern cancer center CEO to board and senior executives

INTRODUCTION

Spending on completed U.S. healthcare construction projects rose from $18 billion in 2003 to $22.6 billion in 2004, according to *Modern Healthcare's* annual construction and design survey (Moon 2005). We are witnessing a healthcare construction boom in the United States to replace aging infrastructure and add capacity that will average approximately $20 billion annually from 2004 to 2010 (Ulrich et al. 2004). Evidence-based design, based on scientific measurement of outcomes associated with facility design initiatives, creates care environments that help patients recover from illnesses and procedures quickly, safely, and with high satisfaction (Berry et al. 2004).

The physical environment inside a hospital is one of the most important and controllable dimensions of patient satisfaction (Fottler et al. 2000). Although every patient interaction represents an opportunity for a hospital to showcase its services, the built environment, also known as the "servicescape":

- contributes to the creation of a healing environment that reflects the relationship between body, mind, and spirit (Linton 2004);
- provides an excellent opportunity to exceed patients' and families' expectations and enhance their feelings of comfort, security, and competent care; and
- fosters a memorable experience that builds the hospital's brand image, provides competitive advantage in the market-place, and allows a hospital to increase its market share.

In addition, healthcare construction projects represent a collaborative opportunity for hospital administrators, physicians, nurses, and allied healthcare professionals to (Fottler et al 2000)

- apply cutting-edge ideas and techniques to diagnosis and treatment (e.g., new imaging technology);
- leverage knowledge obtained from providing direct patient care and observing the reactions of patients and families (e.g., positioning nursing stations and supplies);
- learn from one another about how to deal with the complexity of providing outstanding, cost-effective care (e.g., patient flow); and
- build transparency and trust by making healthcare professionals feel that their input matters and that a shared vision can bridge differences in outlook and training.

As discussed below, a new facility can reduce patient and staff stress, increase patient safety, and improve healthcare outcomes. The purpose of this chapter is to explore the impact of healing design improvements on patient and employee satisfaction, clinical outcomes, and competitive positioning and to emphasize the interdisciplinary collaboration necessary to make effective building improvements.

REDUCING PATIENT STRESS

Healthcare is a needed service that most patients and families dread. Yet, a pleasant environment has been associated with measurable decreases in pain; improved T-cell mediated immunity and natural killer cell activity; and lowered levels of norepinephrine and cortisol, blood-based markers of stress (Rabin 1999). New building materials, such as improved sound-absorbing ceiling tiles, have decreased the stress associated with noise pollution and improved the duration and restfulness of sleep (Ulrich et al. 2004).

Flexible zones that permit family to stay in a patient's room decrease their sense of disruption and increase satisfaction with care (Berry et al. 2004). New hospital construction, which generally increases the number of single rooms, increases patients' sense of privacy. A sense of privacy also is associated with decreased stress and increased satisfaction. A substantial proportion of patients separated from other patients only by curtains reported withholding or refusing part of their medical history because of privacy issues (Ulrich et al. 2004).

IMPROVING STAFF WELL BEING

New hospital construction may be disruptive in the short term, but it sends a long-term message that the health and safety of the workers matter to an organization. More effective air filtration has decreased the number of employee days lost to sick building syndrome. Improved ergonomic design of patient bed areas and nursing work stations decreased back injuries at one hospital 43 percent, from 83 to 47 per 200,000 work hours (Ulrich et al. 2004). Administrators at a newly constructed hospital credit the improved environment with helping them to decrease nursing turnover from 20 percent to 10 percent. The new hospital represented a proactive approach rather than a reactive policy of trying to match a nearby competitor's salary and benefit package (Berry et al. 2004).

Patient safety can enhance worker safety. In a study of errors during residency, 52 percent of errors observed were associated with feelings of diminished self-esteem, and 56 percent of errors might have been prevented with additional knowledge, skills, or improved systems of care (Cohn 1985). Facilities with systems that prevent errors through standardization and improved information capabilities help workers feel proud of the care that they provide and reduce the likelihood of additional errors because the caregiver was thinking about a past error rather than the present patient care situation (Reiling 2004).

IMPROVING SAFETY AND CLINICAL OUTCOMES

Caring for patients involves a complex choreography. Improvements in hospital design can facilitate providing care that is safe, effective, timely, and efficient in a number of ways:

- Decentralized nursing stations with supplies close to the patient's bedside save time walking and allow caregivers to spend more time providing direct patient care (Ulrich et al. 2004).
- Methodist Hospital reduced patient falls by 80 percent in its new hospital by locating toilets closer to the bedside, using double doors to widen entrance to bathrooms, purchasing folding beds that family and staff could wheel into the bathroom to facilitate transfers, and employing an infrared beam to alert nurses when patients climb out of bed (Berry et al. 2004).

- Designing areas for family members to stay in a patient's room increases the likelihood that someone can help a patient at night, when staffing may be thinnest, and prevent falls.
- Building infrastructure to support computerized order entry and medication barcoding eliminates handwriting recognition errors and decreases adverse drug reactions due to allergies and drug interactions; it also decreases the number of calls to physicians, which helps them function more efficiently than when paging disrupts their concentration (Berry et al. 2004).
- Acuity-adaptable rooms with capability for electronic monitoring of cardiac rate, rhythm, blood pressure, and oxygen saturation decrease patient transfers, maintain continuity of care, decrease medication errors, and shorten patients' length of stay (Ulrich et al. 2004). Patient room transfers add an average of 18 non–value added steps, interfere with continuity of care, and add approximately one day to length of stay. Methodist Hospital, which calculated the cost of the 18 steps and the additional length of stay, estimated saving approximately $12 million annually in constructing acuity-adaptable rooms (Berry et al. 2004).
- Single-bed rooms with improved air filtration systems and easily accessible alcohol-based hand-rub dispensers for caregivers' use decreased hospital-acquired pediatric ICU infection rates from an average of 3.62 to 1.87 per patient and shortened average length of stay from 25 to 11 days compared to the previous open-space unit (Ben-Abraham et al. 2002).

Safety design principles stemming from a national conference in April 2002 are summarized in Figure 8.1 (Reiling 2004). They include standardization to minimize variability, automation where possible, and immediate accessibility of information.

Despite construction cost increases due to rapidly rising demand for building materials, budgeted design elements play an important role in the healing process. Natural light can reduce

Figure 8.1: Safety Design Principles

1. Standardization: Checklists for caregivers, especially for high-risk patients and procedures or procedures performed uncommonly:
    *   Preoperative, intraoperative, and postoperative care, especially specialty-specific care (e.g., orthopedic traction)
    *   Administration of medications and blood transfusions
    *   Patients needing restraints
    *   Patients at high risk for falls
    *   Patients at high risk of self-injury (e.g., depression, suicide risk)
    *   Patients who are immunocompromised or anticoagulated
    *   Imaging hazards, for example, transfer of morbidly obese patients
2. Automation, where possible, to reduce human error
3. Scalability and adaptability
4. Close visual proximity of caregivers to patient
5. Real-time accessibility of accurate information
6. Noise reduction
7. Minimization of interruptions and fatigue
8. Involvement of patients and family in care plan
9. Creation and promotion of a safety culture based on
    *   shared values
    *   anticipatory intelligence
    *   informed staff
    *   a blame-free environment that celebrates learning rather than finger pointing
    *   reporting of sentinel events and near misses with after-action reviews conducted without fear of penalty
    *   spirit of collaboration and ongoing improvement

Source: Adapted from Reiling, 2004. Used with permission.

depression, analgesic use, medication costs, and length of stay. Positive distractions, such as healing gardens and views or paintings of nature produce positive emotional and physiologic changes (Ulrich et al. 2004). Environmental satisfaction ranked second only to perceived quality of clinical care as a predictor of overall satisfaction, plans to return to the same hospital for care, and willingness to recommend it to others (Harris et al. 2002).

CASE PRESENTATION

To illustrate the benefits of evidence-based hospital design, Berry et al. (2004) described a case based on experience at multiple healthcare institutions throughout the United States. In this hypothetical construct, the new hospital would represent an institution's core values of superior quality, patient safety, patient-focused care, family friendliness, staff support, cost sensitivity, eco-sustainability, and community responsibility. The design innovations included:

- oversized single rooms (365 square feet) with dedicated space for patient, family, and staff activities and sufficient capacity for in-room procedures;
- maximizing daylight exposure to patient rooms and employee work spaces;
- acuity-adaptable rooms;
- double-door bathroom access;
- decentralized, barrier-free nursing stations that place nurses in close proximity to their patients and supplies; most supplies located in or near patient rooms;
- HEPA filters on all heating, ventilation, and air-conditioning (HVAC) ducts to improve filtration of incoming outside air and to eliminate recirculated air; ultraviolet light at the start of the duct to kill microorganisms;
- alcohol-rub hand hygiene dispensers located at the bedside in each patient room to reduce staff-to-patient transmission of pathogens;
- flexible, adaptable spaces for advanced technology, including operating rooms for robotic surgery, endovascular suites for minimally invasive surgery with sophisticated imaging

capabilities, and diagnostic imaging suites built to support continuous advances in software and hardware;

- computerized order entry and barcode verification technology to minimize medication errors and improve operational efficiency;
- peaceful settings, including displays of nature and artwork, space to listen to music, and gardens to escape the confines of the hospital;
- noise-reducing measures, including sound-absorbing floors and ceilings and a wireless paging system that eliminates overhead paging;
- consultation spaces conveniently located to facilitate conversations between healthcare professionals, patients, and families;
- patient education centers on each floor, offering reading materials, videotapes, and Internet access to disease-specific support groups that can improve understanding of illness; and
- staff support facilities including cafeteria, windowed break rooms with outside access, a day-care facility, and an exercise club.

CASE ANALYSIS

Budgetary Concerns

Although hospitals require design professionals to demonstrate competency in healing environments, few facilities currently achieve that goal. Budgets developed based on historical databases underestimate the long-term savings of transformational design based on innovative planning and evidence-based research. Transformational design is that which enables an organization to function at maximum efficiency and effectiveness, ensures a high level of patient safety, and delivers a care experience that exceeds patients' and families' expectations. A truly transformational facility may cost more to build initially but can also decrease waste, improve operations, cut errors, and achieve significant savings compared to conventional design during the life of the building (Malkin 2005).

The estimated incremental costs for the design improvements mentioned above were nearly recovered within one year, based on reductions in patient falls, decreased need for patient transfers with acuity-adaptable rooms, fewer hospital-acquired infections, reduced usage of pain medicine due to positive distractions, and decreased staff turnover. Additional sources of revenue captured by hospitals that invest in evidence-based design include increased market share and enhanced philanthropic support resulting from donors wanting to be associated with a facility that provides an optimal care experience (Berry et al. 2004).

The Importance of Collaboration

In proposals for new construction, healing environments are mentioned as though they are commodities rather than the result of a systematic, unending approach to improving policies and procedures that put patients' needs first. Physicians and nurses who are with patients and their families daily can have valuable insights into facility design. Their input needs to be sought before plans are drawn up (Fottler et al. 2000).

Physician and nurse champions should be invited to tour other hospital construction projects and brief their colleagues at multiple stages of the planning process to create realistic expectations and to benefit from their colleagues' experience. Listening actively and empathetically to practicing healthcare professionals is a win-win situation for patient care and for the organization (Cohn, Gill, and Schwartz 2005). Collaboration increases the chance that physicians can influence patients and other potential community donors to support the capital campaign and decreases the likelihood of expensive system redesigns once construction is underway.

Many hospital employees and physicians stay longer at a hospital than hospital executives. A newly constructed hospital may be healthcare professionals' second home for longer than the term of the administrative team; thus, it is important to encourage health professionals' feelings of ownership. Salary and benefits are short-term incentives. The quality of the work environment is key to retention and recruitment in the long term.

CONCLUSION

Incorporating evidence-based design improvements contributes to the maintenance of a healing environment and decreases the stress of illness for patients and families. It also represents an opportunity to improve collaboration among healthcare professionals, incorporate new technology, and leverage healthcare professionals' expertise to improve care and the visibility of the hospital within the community.

KEY CONCEPTS

- The business case for design improvement is strong and solidly grounded in carefully gathered evidence.
- Evidence-based design, based on scientific measurement of outcomes associated with facility design initiatives, creates care environments that help patients recover more rapidly, more safely, and with higher satisfaction, thus creating competitive advantage in the marketplace.
- By helping staff care for patients in an improved setting, hospitals send a positive message to healthcare professionals that can facilitate recruitment and retention.
- Although costs may be initially higher for evidence-based design innovations, in most cases, the costs can be recouped

within several years through operational savings and reductions in waste and errors that result in measurable and sustainable long-term benefits.

- Healthcare construction projects represent critical opportunities to derive input from a variety of healthcare professionals, thereby fostering collaboration to improve patient care.

REFERENCES

Ben-Abraham, R, O. Szold, A. Vardi, M. Weinberg, Z. Barzilay, and G. Paret. 2002. "Do Isolation Rooms Reduce the Rate of Nosocomial Infections in a Pediatric Intensive Care Unit?" *Journal of Critical Care* 17 (3): 176–80.

Berry, L.L., D. Parker, R.C. Coile, D.K. Hamilton, D.D. O'Neill, and B.L. Sadler. 2004. "The Business Case for Better Buildings." *Frontiers of Health Services Management* 21 (1): 3–24.

Cohn, K.H. 1985. "Misadventures in Surgical Residency: Analysis of Mistakes During Training." *Current Surgery* 42 (4): 278–85.

Cohn, K.H., S. Gill, and R. Schwartz. 2005. "Gaining Hospital Administrators' Attention: Ways to Improve Physician-Hospital Management Dialogue." *Surgery* 137 (2): 132–40.

Fottler, M.D., R.C. Ford, V. Roberts, and E.W. Ford. 2000. "Creating a Healing Environment: The Importance of the Service Setting in the New Consumer-Oriented Healthcare System." *Journal of Healthcare Management* 45 (2): 91–107.

Harris. P.B., G. McBride, C. Ross, and L. Curtis. 2002. "A Place to Heal: Environmental Sources of Satisfaction Among Hospital Patients. *Journal of Applied Social Psychology* 32 (6): 1276–99.

Linton, P.E. 2004. "Healing Environments: Creating a Total Healing Environment." *Journal of Healthcare Design* 5: 167–74.

Malkin, J. 2005. "Designing a Better Environment." In *Improving Healthcare with Better Building Design*, edited by S.O. Marberry, 109–24. Chicago: Health Administration Press.

Moon, S. 2005. "Construction—and Costs—Going Up." *Modern Healthcare* 35 (10): 30–38.

Rabin, B. 1999. *Stress, Immune Function, and Health*. New York: Wiley-Liss.

Reiling, J. 2004. "Facility Design Focused on Patient Safety. *Frontiers of Health Services Management* 21 (1): 41–46.

Ulrich, R., X. Quan, C. Zimring, A. Joseph, and R. Choudhary. 2004. "The Role of the Physical Environment in the Hospital of the 21st Century: A-Once-in-a-Lifetime Opportunity." [Online report; retrieved 5/4/05.] http://www.healthdesign.org/research/reports/pdfs/role_physical_env.pdf.

CHAPTER 9

Collaborative Opportunities in Disease-Based Care

Kenneth H. Cohn and Murray F. Brennan

> Much of our generation may lament the passing of what is
> embodied in professionalism, but the generation that will
> care for us has already made the transition from entrepre-
> neurship to team orientation.
>
> —*Murray F. Brennan*

INTRODUCTION

Specialization is inevitable because of expanding medical knowledge and public demand. Over time, the question will not be
whether large cities develop disease-based care, but when and in
what form. Disease-based hospitals, trauma centers, cancer centers, and cardiovascular centers incorporate practitioners from multiple disciplines to focus on the management of diseases for which
they have specialized knowledge and experience.

The Institute of Medicine report *Keeping Patients Safe* (2004)
supports interdisciplinary collaboration that is the cornerstone
of disease-based hospital collaboration and points to randomized
trials of more than 1,100 patients that demonstrated decreased
length of stay, better understanding of the care plan, and more
favorable perception of teamwork in settings characterized by

interdisciplinary collaboration. The purpose of this chapter is to examine an integrated sarcoma service as an example of disease-based care, pointing out strengths and concerns that highlight the need for ongoing dialogue and collaboration among health-care professionals.

CASE PRESENTATION

Sarcomas are tumors composed of cancer cells resembling embryonic connective tissue. Treatment requires the multimodal services of surgical specialists, medical oncologists, radiation oncologists, pathologists, nurses, physical therapists, and social workers. They meet formally every week to discuss new patients, monitor existing patients, compile basic demographics, review pathology, and record planned treatment for subsequent outcome analyses. Typical examples that would mandate treatment change would be a diagnosis based on molecular biologic techniques rather than conventional microscopic tissue pathology that changes the cancer diagnostic subtype and hence treatment. A computerized database identifies risk factors such as antecedent radiation exposure and familial disposition. The database tracks complications of therapy, local recurrence, and sites of spread of disease to distant organs, thus facilitating monitoring, outcomes assessment, and evidence-based treatment decisions.

During these meetings, participants also identify patients eligible for entry into ongoing clinical trials to test hypotheses in a data-driven fashion.

CASE ANALYSIS

Rationale for Disease-Based Care

One of the rewarding aspects of caring for a large volume of sarcoma patients is the ability to identify patients who need extensive multidisciplinary care as well as those with an excellent prognosis who are best served by limited operations. This approach has allowed limb-sparing surgery to replace amputation as the primary treatment for patients with sarcomas of the arms and legs without compromising survival (Yang et al. 1998). Life-tables, based on decades of experience, allow specialists to predict the risk of death from sarcoma for individual patients according to tumor size, location, and microscopic pathologic features, as compared to prognosis for a population of cancer patients with similar histopathologic diagnoses (Kattan, Leung, and Brennan 2002).

A comprehensive approach to disease-based care allows healthcare professionals to collaborate **before** patients receive treatment, to determine the diagnosis precisely, and to adopt the latest advances in cancer care by interacting with other specialists. It is a privilege to care for patients, and healthcare professionals have an obligation to do it well, starting with the initial patient encounter. During the physician-patient encounter, healthcare professionals make decisions that can affect patient outcomes for years to come. Therefore, a multidisciplinary, collaborative approach can help to ensure that everyone with expertise has a chance to reflect and listen to other talented healthcare professionals to optimize patient outcomes (Brennan 1996).

Avoiding complications is key to providing cost-effective care (Khuri 2005). The overall cost of care needs to be considered, as well as daily charges in comparing different institutions and care settings. Providing disease-based care requires caring for patients and their families in a comprehensive fashion based on knowledge, availability, competence, and empathy (Brennan 1998).

Another key to providing effective patient care is participation in local and national clinical trials. Success draws additional patients and makes it possible to expand services and hire additional specialists whose employment might not be cost-effective at smaller volumes—specialists such as nurses who facilitate recruitment and treatment of patients in research protocols. Continuing success of disease-focused centers also facilitates recruitment and retention of a variety of other healthcare professionals. Training programs can prepare residents, fellows, nurses, physical therapists, social workers, and physicians from other disciplines to support disease-based care in other locales.

Over the past two decades, disease-focused approaches have flourished due to improved service delivery and improved outcomes. Multiple recent analyses have shown that high-volume institutions have lower operative mortality and better long-term outcomes than lower volume institutions (Lieberman et al. 1995, Begg et al. 1998, Birkmeyer et al. 2003, MacKenzie et al. 2006).

Concerns Regarding Disease-Based Care

Disease-based care calls into question the traditional academic organization into departments and sections. Traditional departments are based on an approach that creates and maintains allegiances based on disciplines, such as surgery or radiation therapy, rather than on disease-based care. A rigid departmental structure discourages interdisciplinary collaboration, allowing fiefdoms to proliferate and interfere with the provision of interdependent care that is safe, effective, patient-centered, timely, efficient, and equitable, in line with the Institute of Medicine recommendations (IOM 2004).

Disease-based care also offers a challenge to the traditional reimbursement approach that often favors procedures over optimal processes and outcomes. Traditional methods of reimbursement can fragment care and lead to an "us versus them" mentality rather than a collaborative approach to care. Perhaps the recent limitations imposed on work hours in residency training will foster a more team-oriented approach as physicians realize that it has become impossible for any specialist acting alone to provide comprehensive care. Incentives that reward a care team rather than individual production also merit consideration.

The model we have described may not apply to all localities. Some tumors are uncommon enough to make it difficult to provide multidisciplinary care in one visit. Patients in rural locations may not want to travel long distances to receive cancer or cardiac care. However, this concern does not obviate the advantages of rural centers analyzing their patient needs and identifying those who would benefit significantly from referral to a major center. Rural surgeons are required to be facile with general surgery, endoscopy, trauma care, and basic orthopedics in an environment with few other colleagues to support them with difficult cases. Training these physicians to identify patients who would benefit from referral for multidisciplinary care is an important aspect of their education.

Telemedicine, including Internet-based consultation, offers an important adjunct for physicians who do not practice in disease-focused settings. An article written in 2003 (Pande et al.) estimated that 250,000 teleconsultations are performed each year and that telementoring is an important part of the telemedicine consultation process. Experts wrote that the main problem limiting widespread diffusion of telemedicine is not lack of technology but lack of an organizational model to capitalize technology that can improve the delivery of healthcare (Scalvini et al. 2004).

Disease-based care confronts challenges of how to care for patients who have complex, comorbid conditions that do not fall into one category, such as the cancer patient who suffers a postoperative heart attack. Clearly, identification of cardiac risk preoperatively is important, as is having sufficient volume to support specialists such as non-invasive cardiologists who have experience at the interface of oncology and heart disease. Disease-based care may encourage the development of new training programs to meet evolving needs. In the interim, strategic collaborative alliances are necessary to ensure that healthcare professionals with needed expertise are readily accessible and available.

Finally, as discussed in Chapter 3 regarding hospitalists, physicians from referral centers need to plan at an early stage for the return of patients to their primary care physicians (PCPs). Termination of therapy can result in considerable anxiety for patients and families if they and their PCPs are not prepared to resume the next phase of care (Cohn 1982).

CONCLUSION

The rigid ordering of care into departments inhibits collaboration by fostering an us-versus-them mentality rather than putting patients and families at the center of the healthcare universe. Recently enacted residency work-hour restrictions and lifestyle considerations of newly trained physicians mandate more collaborative care models focused on patients and their diseases rather than individual disciplines such as radiation therapy or surgery. Strategic collaborative alliances are necessary to ensure accessibility and availability of expertise for patients with complex comorbid conditions.

KEY CONCEPTS

- A multidisciplinary, collaborative approach can help to ensure that everyone with expertise has a chance to reflect and listen to other talented healthcare professionals to optimize patient outcomes.
- The overall cost of care as well as daily charges must be considered in comparing different institutions and care settings; avoiding complications is key to providing cost-effective care.
- Disease-based care helps confront the challenges of caring for patients who have complex, comorbid conditions that do not fall into one category and calls into question the traditional organization into disciplines.
- When professionals collaborate using disease-based care, they can care for patients and their families in a comprehensive fashion based on knowledge, availability, competence, and empathy.

REFERENCES

Begg, C.B., L. Cramer, W.J. Hoskins, and M.F. Brennan. 1998. "Impact of Hospital Volume on Operative Mortality for Major Cancer Surgery." *JAMA* 280 (20): 1747–51.

Birkmeyer, J.D., T.A. Stukel, A.E. Siewers, P.P. Goodney, D.E. Wennberg, and F.L. Lucas. 2003. "Surgeon Volume and Operative Mortality in the United States." *New England Journal of Medicine* 349 (22): 2117–27.

Brennan, M.F. 1996. "The Surgeon as a Leader in Cancer Care: Lessons Learned from the Study of Soft Tissue Sarcoma." *Journal of the American College of Surgeons* 182 (6): 520–29.

———. 1998. "The Surgeon as a Leader in Cancer Care." *Australia and New Zealand Journal of Surgery* 68 (10): 691–97.

Cohn, K.H. 1982. "Chemotherapy from an Insider's Perspective." *Lancet* 1 (8279): 1006–1009.

Institute of Medicine (IOM). 2004. *Keeping Patients Safe: Transforming the Work Environment of Nurses*, 361–63. Washington, DC: National Academies Press.

Kattan, M.W., D.H. Leung, and M.F. Brennan. 2002. "Postoperative Nomogram for 12-Year Sarcoma-Specific Death." *Journal of Clinical Oncology* 20 (3): 791–96.

Khuri, S. 2005. "The NSQIP: A New Frontier in Surgery." *Surgery* 138 (5): 837–43.

Lieberman, M.D., H. Kilburn, M. Lindsey, and M.F. Brennan. 1995. "Relation of Perioperative Deaths to Hospital Volume Among Patients Undergoing Pancreatic Resection for Malignancy." *Annals of Surgery* 222 (5): 638–45.

Mackenzie, E.J., F.P. Rivara, G.J. Jurkovich, A.B. Nathens, K.P. Frey, B.L. Egleston, D.S. Salkever, and D.O. Scharfstein. 2006. "A National Evaluation of Trauma-Center Care on Mortality." *New England Journal of Medicine* 354 (4): 366–78.

Pande, R.U., Y. Patel, C.J. Powers, G. D'ancona, and H.L. Karamanoukian. 2003. "The Telecommunication Revolution in the Medical Field: Present Applications and Future Perspective." *Current Surgery* 60 (6): 636–40.

Scalvini, S., M. Vitacca, L. Paletta, A. Giordano, and B. Balbi. 2004. "Telemedicine: A New Frontier for Effective Healthcare Services." *Monaldi Archives for Chest Disease* 61 (4): 226–33.

Yang, J.C., A.E. Chang, A.R. Baker, W.F. Sindelar, D.N. Danforth, S.L. Topalian, T. DeLaney, E. Glatstein, S.M. Steinberg, M.J. Merino, and S.A. Rosenberg. 1998 "Randomized Prospective Study of the Benefit of Adjuvant Radiation Therapy in the Treatment of Soft Tissue Sarcomas of the Extremity." *Journal of Clinical Oncology* 16 (1): 197–203.

CHAPTER 10

Taking a Proactive, Collaborative Approach to Malpractice Issues

Kenneth H. Cohn, Donald Thieme, and Andrew Feldman

> The malpractice system, by and large, is not about techni-
> cal competence. It's about bad outcomes and, too often,
> bad relationships.
>
> —*A Tennessee pediatrician (Weiss 2005)*

INTRODUCTION

Healthcare professionals may practice at the highest level of competence, implement the latest directives, and still be named in a
malpractice suit. Numerous polls have documented that the fear of
being sued for malpractice is constantly on healthcare professionals' minds and that the current state of malpractice has reached a
crisis in many regions of the United States (Charles 1991, Weiss 2005).

The National Center for State Courts reported an 18 percent
increase in malpractice filings from 1993 to 2002 (Weiss 2005), a
rate that exceeded population growth over the last decade by 5
percent (U.S. Census Bureau 2005). According to the Physician
Insurers Association of America (PIAA), whose member companies insure approximately 60 percent of U.S. physicians in private
practice, the average award for a malpractice conviction has more

than doubled from under $150,000 in 1988 to nearly $330,000 in 2003. Moreover, payments in excess of $1,000,000, which accounted for less than 1 percent of awards in 1988, accounted for over 8 percent of awards in 2003 (Weiss 2005).

Of physicians polled, 72 percent stated that they have limited the scope of their services because of malpractice concerns. In a study of 825 Pennsylvania physicians in high-risk specialties, 92 percent of respondents admitted to ordering tests, diagnostic procedures, or consultations that they did not think were medically necessary (Studdert et al. 2005). Although physicians reported going against their own clinical judgment to minimize their malpractice exposure, they were skeptical that over-ordering improves outcomes. A Pennsylvania obstetrician confessed, "It's sad to step back and realize how much money is being wasted on this. Even the patients are getting tired of so much care, but we all know what will happen if anything goes wrong" (Weiss 2005).

An Ohio family practitioner affirmed, "Let's face it, in malpractice cases, the trouble does not begin with lawyers, it begins … with interactions with patients" (Colon 2002). Under pressure from insurers, physicians are seeing patients for shorter time periods, leaving some patients with the feeling that they are being sent out without their needs being met. New technology, such as CT and MRI scans, takes patients away from physicians and interposes delays until the physicians ordering the tests can obtain and review the reports, which increases patient and family anxiety. The growth of consumerism has created expectations for instant gratification, which current processes have difficulty fulfilling.

Malpractice and its accompanying defensive behavior represent failure of collaboration among healthcare professionals, patients, and families. The growing fear of malpractice and the introduction of proven methods to improve quality and safety provide the opportunity to reduce clinical and legal risk simultaneously. The purpose of this chapter is to discuss malpractice from a proactive and collaborative viewpoint that helps healthcare professionals deliver outstanding outcomes and brings patients, families, and healthcare professionals into closer alignment.

What Is Malpractice?

Malpractice is defined as the failure to exercise the skill, care, and learning expected of a reasonably prudent healthcare provider. The concept of negligence derives from the principle that a person injured through careless actions of another has a moral right to compensation to return the injured person to a situation closer to that person's original state before injury. In general, four elements must pertain to prove negligence (Strasberg 2005a):

1. Acceptance of responsibility for a patient's care
2. Breach of care
3. Patient suffering
4. An injury that occurred as a direct result of a breach of care

The plaintiff's lawyer (Kern 1994) assesses whether the healthcare professional

- disregarded contraindications to treatment,
- failed to advise the patient and family about alternative remedies,
- did not possess the skill and training to provide care, or
- failed to follow specialty guidelines.

Four situations can result in adverse patient outcomes, many of which are preventable with anticipation, training, and improved warning systems: (1) errors in judgment, technique, or oversight; (2) biologic variation in enzyme metabolism that results in idiosyncratic responses; (3) communication failures; (4) systems failures (Wire 2004). The patient safety movement deserves credit for bringing to national attention the concept that poor outcomes may result from poorly designed systems of care (Leape and Berwick 2005; Kohn, Corrigan, and Donaldson 2000). We discuss these concepts further in the following sections.

COLLABORATIVE, PROACTIVE APPROACHES TO MALPRACTICE

In Chapter 4, we discussed the Institute of Medicine recommendation that advocated translating concepts of aviation team training and crew resource management to the healthcare sector to improve patient safety (Grogan et al. 2004). Strasberg (2005b) outlined a rationale to create a culture of safety, using checklists for obtaining informed consent and for delivering preoperative, intraoperative, and postoperative care. He noted that many industries have stopping rules that are applied in the face of dangerous conditions to stop a process before irreparable damage occurs, as in flight rules that divert a plane to another landing field in inclement weather.

The Joint Commission on Accreditation of Healthcare Organizations (JCAHO) recommendations call for a time-out prior to a procedure to verify the patient's name and location of the procedure, review the patient's history and medications, and discuss possible anesthesia concerns (Runy 2005). Additional systems-based responses include removing concentrated electrolyte solutions from nursing stations to prevent fatal medication errors, having one type of medication pump throughout the hospital to limit the number of devices with which nurses must be familiar, and treating patients on anticoagulant medications in dedicated clinics (Leape and Berwick 2005).

Ideally, more widespread adoption of practice guidelines could make it easier to achieve positive outcomes, but the pattern of tort reforms to date has not tied liability law restructuring to systemic, evidence-based changes in medical practice (Budetti 2005). Many physicians have been unwilling to develop guidelines partly because of time pressures, concern that guidelines do not actually improve results (Berry 2004), and fear that failure to follow guidelines will increase litigation (Kern 1994). Physicians have labeled guidelines "cookbook medicine." They quip, "The patient didn't read the book," when they have difficulty making a diagnosis because of variation from textbook symptoms.

Physicians discuss evidence-based medicine in groups such as journal clubs and morbidity and mortality conferences, but implement it as individuals. McGlynn et al. (2003) estimated that only 55 percent of evidence-based preventive and chronic disease services are delivered in the United States due to variation in physician practice, which is a breeding ground for error. Reinertsen and Schellekens (2005) pointed out the paradox of physician autonomy in that as patients suffer injury, physician autonomy is reduced through regulatory and health plan oversight of medical decision making.

A path toward an evidence-based approach could emerge from the patient safety movement but will require further interaction among disparate groups (Budetti 2005). Additional approaches to obtaining improved clinical and emotional outcomes merit consideration, such as captive insurance companies, the 100,000 Lives Campaign, the power of apology, family-driven efforts such as the Josie King Foundation, and positive deviance.

Captive Insurance Companies

A captive insurance company is an organization that is wholly owned by its insured clients. Captive insurance companies usually form to provide self-insurance to larger hospitals and hospital systems. Recently, smaller community hospitals have begun to self-insure. As malpractice premiums rise and become prohibitive for some specialties, community hospitals have created captive insurance companies to insure physicians' practices and prevent services from leaving their hospitals.

The assumption of risk requires a self-insured organization to develop effective internal educational systems and control systems to improve patient care and avoid the financial consequences of malpractice claims. Organizations thus become more motivated to develop guidelines with medical staff before introducing new services and to review strengths and weaknesses of current programs on an ongoing basis.

Field-tested tools are available to improve patient outcomes through risk management programs. The CRICO organization, which covers a number of Harvard affiliated institutions and 9,200 physicians, uses its Risk Management Foundation (www.rmf.harvard.edu) as its loss-prevention manager as well as its claims processor. For obstetrics, the Foundation developed patient and newborn simulators, team-training exercises, and office-practice reviews to reduce the risk of adverse outcomes and claims. Simulations involved clinical scenarios with procedures and videotaped dialogue with patients that practitioners reviewed with experts. The application of proactive programs has reduced the captive insurance company's annual premium for obstetricians from an average of $100,000 to $43,000, approximately 65 percent of current local commercial market rates (CRICO 2005).

The 100,000 Lives Campaign

The Institute for Healthcare Improvement (IHI) began an 18-month campaign in December 2004 to enlist thousands of hospitals across the United States to implement six changes in care that have been proven in case studies to improve patient outcomes and prevent avoidable deaths (Berwick et al. 2006), a common source of malpractice actions (Davis 2005) (See Appendix 10.1 for further details):

1. **Rapid response teams** to decrease unanticipated cardiac arrests and hospitals' overall death rates

2. **Evidence-based care for patients with acute heart attacks,** proven to cut the risk of death from heart attack over 20 percent (Comarow 2005)
3. **Preventing adverse drug events,** implementing medication reconciliation, that is, updating patients' medication lists frequently, decreases medication errors in hospitals that do not have the resources to afford computerized physician order entry, barcoding, and other expensive technology (Comarow 2005)

The final three recommendations involve limiting or preventing hospital acquired infections, which are implicated in the deaths of approximately 90,000 patients annually in the United States:

4. **Preventing infections in central venous lines,** estimated to cause 14,000 to 28,000 deaths per year in hospitalized U.S. patients (IHI 2005b)
5. **Preventing surgical site infections,** which complicate an estimated 780,000 operations per year in the United States (Comarow 2005)
6. **Improving outcomes in patients receiving mechanical ventilation** and preventing ventilator-associated pneumonia, which carries a mortality rate over 40 percent (IHI 2005d)

A nurse commented, "I have been a nurse for 20 years and no one ever held up zero bad outcomes as a goal.... It's a whole new way of looking at our jobs" (IHI 2005d). Another ICU nurse reinforced the importance of multidisciplinary collaboration to achieve outstanding outcomes: "There is no single key to implementing the strategies. It takes hard work, surveillance, cheerleading, education, and continuous assessment and monitoring (IHI 2005e).

Dr. Richard Shannon, chairman of medicine at Allegheny General Hospital, reached a similar conclusion from his work with the Pittsburgh Regional Health Institute (PRHI) described in Chapter 5: "[W]e can make a difference, we can change this. I believe that if we eliminated medical errors there would be no malpractice. I now believe, through PHRI, eliminating medical errors is entirely possible, but the work begins with us. The work begins at the patient's bedside. *The work begins in collaboration with the people that provide the care. The work begins by listening to what they know about how to make things better, not the historical top-down approach"* (Savary and Crawford-Mason 2006).

The Power of Apology

When adverse outcomes occur, despite the best intentions and systems of care, healthcare professionals must acknowledge the outcome, as outlined in JCAHO 2001 standards (Wire 2004). Patients especially value knowing why an error happened and how recurrences will be prevented, information that demonstrates a lesson has been learned (Gallagher and Levinson 2005).

Caregivers historically have tended to refrain from admitting error because they feared medicolegal consequences. Leape (2005) has added that additional reasons include the emotional challenge of admitting error, lack of awareness of how silence upsets patients, and lack of formal training in communication of errors. He cited research that an apology is an essential part of care after a patient has been harmed and that many malpractice cases result from patients and families being angry when physicians and hospitals refuse to talk with them in a straightforward way. He advocated a four-part approach:

1. Acknowledge the event.
2. Provide an explanation of what went wrong; be careful not to hide behind medical jargon.
3. Show remorse.
4. Make amends.

The Sorry Works! Coalition (2005) is a nationwide organization of physicians, lawyers, insurers, and patient advocates that was launched in February 2005 to promote full disclosure and apologies for medical errors as a middle-ground solution to the medical liability crisis: fewer lawsuits and medical errors and swifter acknowledgement of and compensation for errors.

The process involves healthcare professionals performing a root-cause analysis and, if the standard of care was not met, meeting with the patient's family to apologize, explain what happened and what they will do differently, and make an offer of settlement. Even if the standard of care was met, hospital officials and the physician meet with the family to explain what happened and answer all questions. This process restores the doctor-patient relationship and improves communication and trust between all parties. The "honesty dividend" reduces the filing of non-meritorious claims and allows healthcare professionals to apologize, learn from errors, and reduce future errors via improvements in systems of care (Sorry Works! Coalition 2005).

The largest medical malpractice insurer in Colorado, COPIC (2005), began a program called "3Rs," for Recognize, Respond, and Resolve, which encourages physicians to respond immediately, apologize to patients who have suffered an adverse outcome, and describe in detail what went wrong. The insurer compensated patients who did not file a lawsuit for expenses including out-of-pocket expenses for follow-up medical care (up to $25,000) and lost time from work ($100/day up to $5,000). Since 2000, COPIC has reported a 50 percent decrease in malpractice claims against their 1,800 physicians and a 23 percent drop in settlement costs.

The Lexington VA Hospital dropped its average payout from $98,000 to $16,000 and the number of lawsuits going to trial through a similar program based on openness and apology. In addition, the University of Michigan Hospital System halved the number of lawsuits and reduced litigation costs from $65,000 to $35,000 per case, saving approximately $2 million per year by adopting a similar program of openness and apology (Sorry Works! Coalition 2005).

"Sorry" works because it addresses the causes of the medical liability crisis by improving collaboration within the inside culture of physician-hospital relations, as opposed to tort reform that tinkers with the outside culture of lawyers, judges, and juries (Wojcieszak 2005). Unlike tort reform, which increases the difficulty of filing and winning large lawsuits, the Sorry Works! approach seeks to make lawsuits unnecessary. The heretofore used "deny and defend approach" makes doctors and hospitals sitting ducks for lawsuits because patients and families grow angry when nobody answers their questions. Polk (2005) wrote, "Transparency … can become the ultimate expression of patient advocacy. It is not a matter of can or should; it is a matter of must."

Family-Driven Efforts: The Josie King Foundation

The Josie King Foundation (2005) represents a way that families can collaborate with healthcare professionals to direct their grief toward improving healthcare for future patients. Josie King died at 18 months as a result of medical errors at Johns Hopkins Medical Center. Her parents created a patient safety program in 2002 to identify safety concerns, revise medical training, focus on proactive safety measures, and empower families to partner in their loved ones' care. The key to such an endeavor lies in understanding the causes of system error so that healthcare professionals can prevent errors from occurring. In their ongoing work with the Foundation, Johns Hopkins has established a policy to encourage adverse event reporting and to prescribe how to communicate errors to patients and families.

Positive Deviance

Finally, positive deviance (PD) is an approach to organizational change based on the premise that solutions to problems already exist within the community. It encompasses intentional behaviors that depart from the norms of a group *in honorable ways* (Weber 2005a). Positive deviance seeks to identify and optimize existing resources to solve problems rather than using the more conventional identification of needs and obtaining of external resources to meet those needs. Keys to the PD method include (Weber 2005a):

- self-identification as a community by members of the community; that is, people see themselves as alike rather than conflicting;
- mutual designation of a problem by the community members, a bottom-up rather than a top-down approach;
- a search for community members on the leading edge who have managed to surmount a problem;
- analysis of meritorious behaviors that enable outliers (positive deviants) to achieve success; and
- introduction and adoption of new behaviors into group practice.

The following case study will show how a community hospital applied the principles of PD to improve collaboration within its healthcare system (Weber 2005b).

CASE PRESENTATION

Waterbury Hospital Health Center is a 234-bed Connecticut community teaching hospital that invited Jerry Sternin to speak at grand rounds in autumn of 2004. As the staff discussed the application of PD to healthcare settings, they identified communication as their most pervasive challenge. Dr. Anthony Cusano, a nephrologist, recalled several post-discharge medication problems that he had dealt with as a member of the hospital's pharmacy and therapeutics committee that resulted from communication lapses. He and nurse Bonnie Sturtevant designed a telephone survey to learn whether recently discharged patients were following their prescribed regimens successfully.

To their surprise, 80 percent of patients were taking their medications incorrectly. For example, one patient, told to take a pill every other day, took it only Tuesday and Thursday, incorrectly assuming that weekends did not count. Another patient, sent home with a variety of new prescriptions, did not take a necessary medication he already had at home because he did not receive a new prescription for it. Additional patients did not fill a prescription because of expense, but did not inform their physicians and thus never learned of alternatives that could have been more affordable.

Nurses who were making the phone calls found the results so startling and the corrective process so satisfying that they told colleagues, who volunteered to make phone calls to recently discharged patients. Within a few months, they had reached over 150 patients and expanded the calling process to include new interns and residents. Dr. Cusano beamed, "They'll be trained to do this from the start … so there'll be a whole generation of doctors out there who'll think this is just the way medicine is done. And it really isn't that difficult. Here you have a window for mistakes that is easy to close. The solution is right there in front of you. But until you see it, you don't know it" (Weber 2005b).

CASE ANALYSIS

Prior to the intervention, Waterbury Hospital readmitted two patients per month on average for failure to adhere to their post-discharge medication plans (Weber 2005b). Dr. Cusano summed up the results to date in the spring of 2005 (Plexus Institute 2005):

The patients getting the calls love to know that someone cares about them, and it makes the staff feel good about what they are doing. We have a team that's been working on finding a good long-term solution, and we realized that people who were getting the calls were close to 100 percent on doing the right things. It turns out that the phone call itself is the solution. So we had to find a way of getting it done for everyone, but it also turns out that the math works: If everyone on staff makes one phone call a month, we can contact every discharged patient. Collecting the information created an interesting paradox. But it makes a lot of sense. If communication is the issue, positive deviance showed us that it is also the answer. To me, this was a beautiful thing.

The power of PD lies in its bottom-up process. Community members rather than the CEO determine where to direct their efforts. They invest effort in figuring out which approaches will yield the best results. Sternin felt that organizational resistance to identifying and following other institutions' best practices was similar to transplant rejection in that it stimulated more conflict than collaboration (Weber 2005a). As with the structured dialogue process described in Chapter 1, what healthcare professionals discover for themselves, they own (Weber 2005b).

CONCLUSION

Proactive, collaborative approaches to malpractice complement tort reform. Positive deviance may succeed where other efforts have failed because it is often easier for groups to change their thinking through action than to implement action based on new ways of thinking. Similarly, the assumption of risk by captive insurance companies requires self-insured organizations to develop effective internal education systems. The 100,000 Lives Campaign represents another grassroots organization of thousands of hospitals to improve outcomes and prevent avoidable complications like hospital-acquired infections and deaths from unanticipated cardiac arrests that can be the source of lawsuits. Finally, Sorry Works! and other coalitions have demonstrated the power of apology to mitigate family anger and demonstrate that caregivers are capable of listening, reflecting, and learning.

KEY CONCEPTS

Effective communication and collaboration:

- Facilitate sharing of information in a timely fashion that may prevent adverse outcomes or limit their scope
- Improve the quality of the practice environment not only for patients and families but also for physicians, nurses, and administrators
- Help patients and families feel that their concerns matter
- Defuse anger and hostility in the event of an undesirable outcome

APPENDIX 10.1 THE SIX STEPS IN THE 100,000 LIVES CAMPAIGN

1) Rapid response teams: These teams were pioneered in Australia and at University of Pittsburgh Medical Center, where they are credited with decreasing unanticipated cardiac arrests and hospitals' overall death rates. The underlying principle is that patients often exhibit signs and symptoms of instability for hours prior to a cardiac arrest and that a team experienced in critical care can rescue patients before irreversible damage occurs. Nurses are encouraged to call the team not only for changes in the patient's pulse, breathing, blood pressure, urine output, and mental status, but also if the nurse has a gut feeling that a patient does not look right. The team is typically composed of an intensive care nurse, respiratory therapist, and hospital physician. After instituting this collaborative program that affirms and strengthens nurses' bedside skills, participating hospitals report 5 to 65 calls per month, with an average drop in cardiac arrests by one-third (IHI 2005a) and a 30-percent drop in unexpected hospital deaths (Srikameswaran 2005).

2) *Evidence-based care for patients with acute heart attacks:* Recommendations include aspirin and beta-blockers on arrival to the hospital, procedures to open up blocked coronary arteries within two hours of arrival, smoking cessation counseling, and prescriptions for aspirin, beta-blockers, and anti-hypertensive drugs on discharge. A large RAND study published in 2003 documented only 40-to-60-percent hospital compliance on average with these measures that have been proven to cut the risk of death from heart attack over 20 percent (McGlynn 2003).

3) *Preventing adverse drug events:* Implementing medication reconciliation requires a clean, accurate list of medications to accompany a patient and be updated continually as the patient moves from admission through discharge. At one participating hospital, the number of adverse drug events dropped from 3.5 to 1 per 1,000 doses within two years after implementation. This reduction is important because medication errors are implicated in 7,000 unnecessary deaths annually in the United States, and medication reconciliation can be performed in hospitals that do not have the resources to afford computerized physician order entry, barcoding, and other expensive technology (Comarow 2005).

4) *Preventing infections in central venous lines:* IHI recommends a five-step approach to decrease catheter-related bloodstream infections, estimated to cause 14,000 to 28,000 deaths per year in hospitalized U.S. patients (IHI 2005b):

a. Hand-washing prior to insertion

b. Using maximal barrier precautions, including sterile gloves, gown, and drapes as well as surgical masks

c. Chlorhexidine rather than iodine-based solutions to disinfect the skin

d. Appropriate site selection and post-placement care, avoiding areas that become contaminated, such as the neck and groin, whenever possible

e. Daily review of line necessity, with prompt removal of lines that are no longer necessary

5) *Preventing surgical site infections:* IHI recommends a four-step approach:

a. Timing perioperative antibiotic dosage so that patients receive preoperative antibiotics approximately 30 minutes prior to incision to permit adequate concentration in skin and subcutaneous tissues, and so that antibiotics are discontinued within 24 hours after surgery to avoid antibiotic resistance

b. Avoiding razors that irritate skin and increase risk of infection

c. Close monitoring of blood sugar, especially in diabetics undergoing heart surgery

d. Maintaining body temperature during surgery at 36 to 38 degrees Celsius

Within a year after implementing the above recommendations, Baptist Hospital in Memphis, Tennessee, decreased its OB-GYN wound infection rate from 1.4 percent to 0.4 percent. Benefis Healthcare in Great Falls, Montana, decreased its infection rate in patients undergoing coronary bypass from 8 percent to 1.2 percent (IHI 2005c).

6) *Improving outcomes in patients receiving mechanical ventilation:* The IHI recommends a four-step approach to all ventilated patients:

1. Raise the head of the bed to an angle of 30 to 45 degrees, 24 hours a day
2. Assess patients' ability to breathe on their own daily, without sedation, for a brief interval
3. Provide medication to lower stomach acidity and decrease the risk of ulcers and bleeding
4. Decrease the risk of blood clots in the legs by intermittent mechanical compression devices or anticoagulants Ventilator-associated pneumonia (VAP) adds, on average, $40,000 to the cost of hospital admission. Up to 46 percent of patients who develop VAP do not survive their hospital stay. Since it began monitoring and enforcing compliance with the aforementioned four steps, Swedish Medical Center has decreased its incidence of VAP from an average of three cases per month to zero since October 2004 (IHI 2005e).

REFERENCES

Berry, W. 2004. "Surgical Malpractice: Myths and Realities." [Online article; retrieved 12/18/05.] http://www.rmf.harvard.edu/patientsafety/forum/default.asp.

Berwick, D.M., D.R. Calkins, C.J. McCannon, and A.D. Hackbarth. 2006. "The 100,000 Lives Campaign: Setting a Goal and a Deadline for Improving Health Care Quality." *JAMA* 295 (3): 324–27.

Budetti, P.P. 2005. "Tort Reform and the Patient Safety Movement: Seeking Common Ground." *JAMA* 293 (21): 2660–62.

Charles, S.C. 1991. "The Psychological Trauma of a Medical Malpractice Suit: A Practical Guide." *Bulletin of the American College of Surgeons* 76 (11): 22–26.

Colon, V.F. 2002. "10 Ways to Reduce Medical Malpractice Exposure." *Physician Executive* 28 (2): 16–18.

Comarow, A. 2005. "Saving Lives: Hospitals Have Signed on to a Six-Part Plan to Avoid a Multitude of Unnecessary Deaths." *U.S. News & World Report*, July 18. .

COPIC. 2005. "Apologies Gain Momentum." [Online article; retrieved 9/27/05.] http://callcopic.com/publications/3rs/3rs_newsletter.htm

CRICO Obstetrics Risk Reduction Program. 2005. [Online article; retrieved 12/18/05.] http://www.rmf.harvard.edu/crico_services/lossprevention/obincentive/default.asp.

Davis, T. 2005. "100,000 Lives Campaign Adds 1,700 Hospitals ... and Counting." *Physician Executive* 31 (3): 20–23.

Gallagher, T.H., and W. Levinson. 2005. "Disclosing Harmful Errors to Patients: A Time for Professional Action." *Archives of Internal Medicine* 165 (16): 1819–24.

Grogan, E.L., R.A. Stiles, D.J. France, T. Speroff, T.A. Morris, B. Nixon, F.A. Gaffney, R. Seddon, and C.W. Pinson. 2004. "The Impact of Aviation-Based Teamwork Training on the Attitudes of Health-Care Professionals." *Journal of the American College of Surgeons* 199 (6): 843–48.

Institute for Healthcare Improvement (IHI). 2005a. "Rapid Response Teams: The Case for Early Intervention." [Online article; retrieved 10/8/05.] http://www.ihi.org/IHI/Topics/CriticalCare/IntensiveCare/ImprovementStories/.

———. 2005b. "Putting Safety on the (Central) Line." [Online article; retrieved 10/8/05.] http://www.ihi.org/IHI/Topics/CriticalCare/IntensiveCare/Literature/.

———. 2005c. "The Steps to Safer Surgery." [Online article; 10/8/05.] http://www.ihi.org/IHI/Topics/PatientSafety/SurgicalSiteInfections/ImprovementStories/.

———. 2005d. "Breathing Safely in the ICU." [Online article; retrieved 10/8/05.] http://www.ihi.org/IHI/Topics/CriticalCare/IntensiveCare/ Literature/.

———. 2005e. "Pursuing Perfection: Report from Health Partners Regions Hospital on Reducing Hospital-Acquired Infection." [Online article; retrieved 10/8/05.] http://www.ihi.org/IHI/Topics/CriticalCare/IntensiveCare/ ImprovementStories/.

Kern, K.A. 1994. "Medicolegal Perspectives on Laparoscopic Bile Duct Injuries." *Surgical Clinics of North America* 74 (4): 979–84.

Kohn, L., J. Corrigan, and M. Donaldson, (eds.). 2000. *To Err Is Human: Building a Safer Health System*. Committee on Quality of Healthcare in America and Institute of Medicine. Washington, DC: National Academies Press.

Josie King Foundation. 2005. [Online home page; retrieved 11/24/05.] http://www.josieking.org.

Leape, L.L., and D.M. Berwick. 2005. "Five Years After *To Err Is Human*: What Have We Learned?" *JAMA* 293 (19): 2384–90.

Leape, L.L. 2005. "Time Has Come to Apologize." [Online article; retrieved 7/2/05.] http://www.rmf.harvard.edu/patientsafety/apologylecturepost.asp.

McGlynn, E.A., S.M. Asch, J. Adams, J. Keesey, J. Hicks, J. DeCristofaro, and E.A. Kerr. 2003. "The Quality of Health Care Delivered to Adults in the United States." *New England Journal of Medicine* 348 (26): 2635–45.

McGlynn, E.A. 2003. "The First National Report Card on Quality of Health Care in America." [Online article; retrieved 5/4/06.] http://www.rand.org/pubs/research_briefs/RB9053-2/index1.html#top.

Plexus Institute. 2005. "A Paradox: Communication is the Issue and the Answer." *Complexity Post* [Online article; created 5/19/05; retrieved 5/23/05.] http://www.plexusinstitute.org/NewsEvents/show_Thursday_Complexity_Posts.cfm?id=127.

Polk, H.C. 2005. "Presidential Address: Quality, Safety, and Transparency." *Annals of Surgery* 242 (3): 293–301.

Reinertsen, J., and W. Schellekens. 2005. *10 Powerful Ideas for Improving Patient Care*, 36–37. Chicago: Health Administration Press.

Runy, L.A. 2005. "25 Things You Can Do to Save Lives Now." *Hospital and Health Networks* 79 (4): 40–48.

Savary, L.M., and C. Crawford-Mason. 2006. *The Nun and the Bureaucrat: How They Found a Simple, Elegant Solution to a Deadly National Healthcare Problem*, 181. Washington, DC: CCM Productions, Inc.

Sorry Works! Coalition. 2005. [Online article; retrieved 5/4/06.] http://www.sorryworks.net/WhatIs.phtml.

Srikameswaran, A. 2005. "Teams Quicken Response in Medical Emergencies." [Online article; retrieved 10/8/05.] http://www.post-gazette.com/pg/05198/538715.stm.

Strasberg, S.M. 2005a. "Biliary Injury in Laparoscopic Surgery: Part 1. Processes Used in Determination of Standard of Care in Misidentification Injuries." *Journal of the American College of Surgeons* 201 (4): 597–603.

———. 2005b. "Biliary Injury in Laparoscopic Surgery: Part 2: Changing the Culture of Cholecystectomy." *Journal of the American College of Surgeons* 201 (4): 604–11.

Studdert, D.M., M.M. Mello, W.M. Sage, C.M. DesRoches, J. Peugh, K. Zapert, and T.A. Brennan. 2005. "Defensive Medicine Among High-Risk Specialist Physicians in a Volatile Malpractice Environment." *JAMA* 293 (21): 2609–17.

U.S. Census Bureau. 2005. "USA QuickFacts State & Country QuickFacts." [Online article; retrieved 12/16/05.] http://QuickFacts.census.gov/qfd/states/00000.html.

Weber, D.O. 2005a. "Positive Deviance, Part 1." *Hospital and Health Networks* [Online article; created 8/14/05; retrieved 10/9/05.] http://www.hhnmag.com.

————. 2005b. "Positive Deviance, Part 2." *Hospital and Health Networks.* [Online article; retrieved 10/9/05.] http://www.hhnmag.com.

Weiss, G.G. 2005. "Malpractice: How Fear Changes Practice." *Medical Economics* [Online article; retrieved 5/7/05.] http://www.memag.com/memag/article/articleDetail.jsp?id=154646.

Wire, K. 2004. "Embracing Poor Outcomes: A Comprehensive Claim Reduction Strategy." In *West's Health Law Handbook*, vol. II, edited by A. Gosfield, 1–38. St. Louis, MO: West Publishing Co.

Wojcieszak, D. 2005. "Medical Malpractice: There Really Is Middle Ground for a Solution." [Online article; retrieved 11/19/05.] http://www.sorryworks.net/media33.phtml.

CHAPTER 11

Building Community and Collaboration with Blogs

Kenneth H. Cohn, Glen Mohr, and Bill Ives

The blog proved to be an invaluable tool for our Medical Advisory Panel. The backbone of the blog was a summary of each meeting in outline form that was posted within a day of each meeting. The blog facilitated our work by providing a convenient platform for continuation of the discussion. Members who couldn't attend a particular meeting could stay informed. It was particularly useful when it came time to write the summary report. Having this organizational tool allowed me to recognize important themes that were relevant to the majority of the medical staff.

—*Medical Advisory Panel cochair*

INTRODUCTION

As mentioned in Chapter 5, physicians are becoming increasingly disaggregated. The failure of reimbursement to keep up with rising expenses has forced many practitioners to increase the volume of patients they see and treat, thereby limiting their time for activities other than direct patient contact and curtailing time for referrals and referring physicians. Currently, some primary care providers do not set foot inside hospitals except to make social visits or to be patients themselves, as discussed in Chapter 3. These changes are a barrier not only to collegiality but also to discussion and reflection on patients with complex, multisystem health issues for whom the written chart may not reflect the entire picture. Inadequate communication can lead to overuse and unnecessary repetition of diagnostic testing. It can also lead to missed opportunities for collaboration and innovation in treatment.

New web technologies offer simple and convenient ways for clinicians to share information, find others who have the information they need, and keep in contact with one another. The purpose of this chapter is to discuss the use of blogs and aggregators to create virtual medical communities.

WHAT IS A "BLOG?"

A blog (short for weblog) is an easily maintained website that allows a group of geographically disconnected people to form a virtual community. A blog makes communicating simple and convenient by allowing new information to be added easily, archiving everything in a permanent, searchable database, and automatically notifying subscribers when new information is added. For overworked healthcare professionals who have neither the time nor the will to learn new software, a blog is user-friendly and can be customized to suit the needs and technological aptitude of the users. Blogs offer significant advantages over e-mail and other common forms of information sharing.

Blogs Simplify Communication

Adding content (posting) to a blog can be as easy as sending an e-mail or making a single click while surfing the Internet. When posting, the author does not have to input a list of e-mail addresses or worry about sending to the entire group information that will interest only some members. By assigning the post to a category or including specific keywords, the author can be certain that those who want the information will receive it. Blogs alert readers to new information either via e-mail or by the more powerful method called "Really Simple Syndication" (RSS) (see Sidebar 11.1).

Blogs Create a Searchable and Instantly Accessible Archive

Everything published on a blog can be readily accessed using a search engine that can find any word in the document rapidly. Once someone answers a question on a blog, the answer becomes part of a permanent searchable knowledge base. Every post and every comment is automatically assigned its own web address (uniform resource locator [URL], also called a permalink). This feature eliminates the need to send the same message multiple times.

Blogs Encourage Transparency

The search capability built into the blog means that each user does not need to maintain a personal archive of e-mail messages. Information that would normally reside in individual hard drives or e-mail in-boxes is available to all members of the community. By facilitating interaction, blogs invite participation and break down silos and hierarchies. New members can get up to speed quickly and begin receiving the information they need by subscribing and searching the archive.

Blogs Enable Secure Centralized Management

Blogging platforms allow an administrator to control access to what is published on a blog. The best platforms allow permissions to be defined specifically as to what individual users can see and

Sidebar 11.1: What is an Aggregator?

Blogs, and a rapidly increasing number of websites such as the *New York Times* (newyorktimes.com) and specialized information sources such as MedScape, generate "RSS feeds," which are streams of messages sent out whenever content is added or changed. An aggregator (also called a "newsreader") is a software tool that enables readers to "subscribe" to feeds.

Like TiVo for the Internet, once an aggregator is set up, it works in the background searching, collecting, filtering, and categorizing. When a user needs information, the aggregator has the information already queued up and organized. This feature enables readers to use information more efficiently by eliminating the time and distraction of logging onto and searching multiple websites and by reducing e-mail traffic.

The most important feature of aggregators is that they allow publishers and readers to connect on an ongoing basis. Where previously the subscription model was limited to institutional publishers, now individuals can subscribe to other individuals' postings. Once a person finds a valuable source of information—for example, another clinician writing about cases that mirror her own—she can subscribe to that "publisher" so that each time the publisher writes something new, the subscriber receives it automatically (Mohr 2005).

who can read individual articles. The utility of blogs in facilitating a clinical priority-setting process is outlined in the following case study.

CASE PRESENTATION

A 750-bed Western hospital system began a structured dialogue process to engage physicians in setting clinical priorities for the next three to five years as it planned the construction of a new hospital that would consolidate two campuses. A medical advisory panel (MAP) was formed of 16 clinically active physicians who committed to attending weekly meetings in return for a commitment from hospital leaders to give serious consideration to implementing the MAP recommendations, as described in Chapter 1. The MAP heard presentations from physicians in all major clinical areas on their recommendations to improve care for the community and foster better physician-physician and physician-administrator communication and collaboration. The MAP collated the recommendations into a consensus report that highlighted the need for major improvement initiatives involving information technology, radiology, the operating room, and the intensive care unit.

A password-protected blog was created to support the structured dialogue process. To make it user-friendly, the blog design included pre-set content categories for presenter reports, meeting minutes, and implementation status. It also included links to common tasks such as adding content and downloading materials. A blog administrator was trained and charged with regularly updating the blog, maintaining the flow of discussion, and ensuring that the blog discussion was integrated with weekly face-to-face meetings. An aggregator facilitated seeking outside sources of information and bringing them into the structured dialogue process. Throughout the process, a physician-facilitator monitored use of the blog, customized the functionality to serve the panelists' needs, and coached the blog administrator.

In the first month of the structured dialogue process, panelists learned how to use the blog during a 20-minute presentation that explained:

1. the blog's purpose in supporting the structured dialogue process and saving physicians' time;
2. examples of how blogs have been used in other healthcare organizations (see Appendix 11.1); and
3. the log-in procedure, likely tasks, and how to obtain technical support.

The blog facilitated the structured dialogue process at every step, as explained below and in Figure 11.1.

The blog provided a convenient distribution point for material relevant to physician presenters and their reports. Medical advisory panel members could download material that explained the structured dialogue process and the criteria that reports were expected to address, which could be sent to physician presenters in their department. When presenters submitted their reports, the reports were uploaded to the blog, which generated an automatic e-mail linking to the report on the blog and reminded panelists to read the reports prior to the weekly MAP meeting.

Within two days after each MAP meeting, minutes were posted to the blog, which helped panelists keep track of what they had done. A calendar maintained on the blog kept important details from being overlooked.

As presentations drew to a close, the blog's search engine facilitated report writing. A large amount of data accumulated in the course of the MAP meetings, which were held weekly for 8 months and comprised over 40 presentations. Panelists could search the archive to find recurring themes and specific comments and examples that otherwise might have faded in memory or have been too time-consuming to locate in the minutes and reports.

The blog also served as the location to post drafts of the MAP report to allow panelists to provide important feedback at a time that was convenient for each panelist.

Building Solidarity and Community

The blog permitted panelists to interact outside the confines of weekly meetings as new ideas surfaced and new issues appeared. The secure, password-protected site allowed panelists to discuss what was on their minds without fear of outsiders reading their comments.

The 24/7 access decreased barriers to participation and allowed even reticent panel members to contribute to the structured dia-

Figure 11.1 Weblog Facilitation of the Structured Dialogue Process

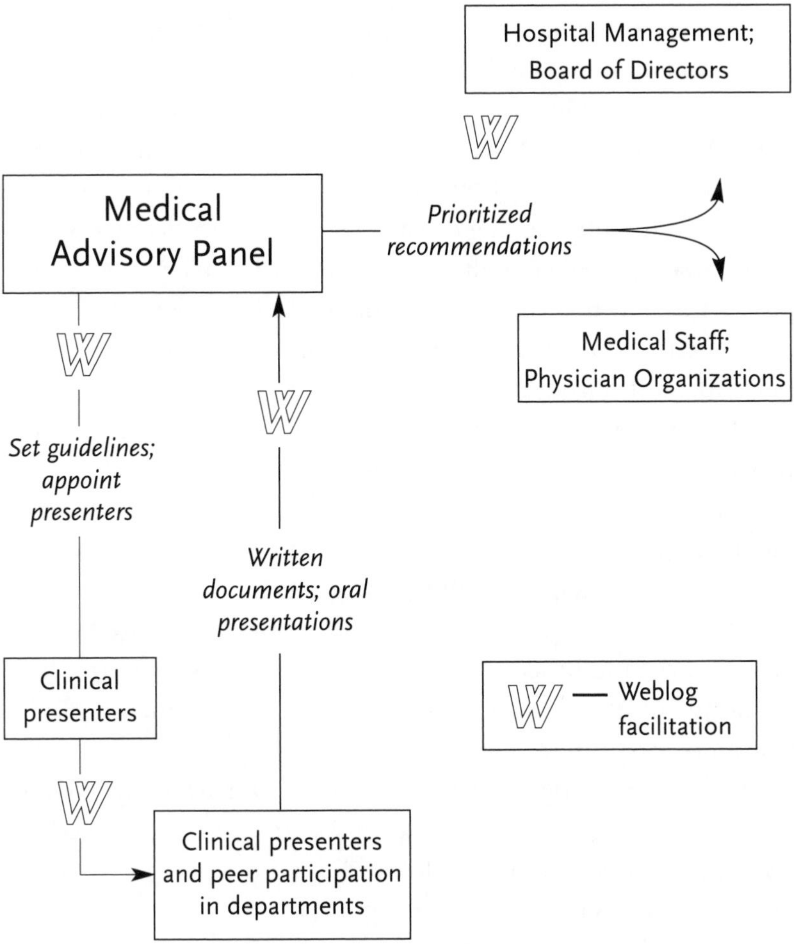

Source: Adapted from the American College of Physician Executives. Cohn, 2002.

logue process. Some panelists found it easier to reflect over weekends than during Monday morning meetings. The blog provided a way to capture their insights. For example, after spending a frustrating weekend on call, a physician panelist posted a detailed log of the time he wasted in radiology trying to access studies of critically ill patients on whom he was consulted. His comments focused the MAP's attention on radiology service issues early in the process and gave others an opportunity to reflect on time they had wasted searching for imaging studies on their patients. One participant commented, "I thought it was just me."

When a department of radiology presentation became a contentious source of differences between physicians and hospital administration, the blog functioned as an after-action review, providing a forum for ongoing discussion. The forum clearly evolved as physicians posted content and comments. The blog also allowed physicians who missed a meeting because of vacation, illness, or a conference to remain current and thus allowed the process to move forward during the summer.

The blog encouraged members to contribute information that they found relevant without worrying about wasting scarce meeting time. Some physicians used the blog to provide outside reading for fellow panelists, for example, an article on differences in cost of care between the United States and Canada.

Because successive drafts of the final report were posted to the blog, the writing process became transparent and supported the development of a consensus report, in which all panelists could take an ownership role.

In short, the blog allowed the MAP to pursue a data-driven consensus approach to clinical priority setting and lowered barriers to participation. When polled at the end of the report-writing process, panelists unanimously endorsed continuation of the blog into the implementation phase and have asked hospital executives to become part of the blog community by extending them passwords to the site.

CASE ANALYSIS

Although blog technology is user-friendly and intuitive, planning carefully its introduction, management, and support is still critical. Healthcare settings require compliance with the Health Insurance Portability and Accountability Act (HIPAA) (Robeznieks 2005). A proactive but flexible organizational policy regarding blog use that encourages informal communication and discourages leaks of proprietary information and patient health information is necessary to foster spontaneity and serendipity. The following four general conditions are necessary for blogs to thrive (Ives and Watlington 2005):

1. The community has a need to document and share information.
2. A bottom-up, decentralized process is already in place or is being developed.
3. A leader or sponsor is committed to integrating the blog into all major functions and processes.
4. The community supports free expression of ideas, especially ideas that do not mesh with current models.

The design and approach employed in the case study ensured that panelists clearly understood the purpose of the blog and how it could facilitate the structured dialogue process. In addition, responsive support not only handled technical issues but, more importantly, monitored use of the blog and adjusted the design and functionality to serve members' evolving needs. For example, initial use of the blog was limited to distributing presenter reports and meeting minutes. Later, new categories were added for implementation notes and links to the final report drafts.

Figure 11.2 lists the lessons learned about employing blogs in medical settings, including keeping expectations realistic, simplifying the user interface, and ensuring that technical support is readily available at times convenient to physicians' usage patterns. Figure 11.3 lists potential uses of blogs in medical settings including to break down silos, complete project management tasks on schedule, and develop virtual physician networks.

Figure 11.2: Recommendations for Using Blogs in Medical Settings

- Keep initial promises and expectations realistic: Physicians are drawn to new processes that allow them to use time more efficiently and effectively and that help them improve processes of care.
- Be explicit about who has access to minimize concerns about confidentiality.
- Do as much setup as possible for the users (for example, assign usernames and passwords rather than requiring them to register) to speed their time to productive use.
- Simplify the user interface as much as possible—resist adding features until they are necessary or users demand them. In the case study, features and categories were not added to the blog until panelists were familiar with the basics of looking at minutes and downloading presenter reports.
- Have a technical support person available who can answer questions without making participants feel stupid.
- Designate and train a specific person to maintain the blog. This person should post regularly and consistently, for example, uploading meeting minutes. In addition, this person should create links and categories to organize data. Most importantly, this person should ensure that dialogue that is on the blog is integrated into face-to-face dialogue.
- Start early to use blog, for example, at the beginning of the structured dialogue process, and incorporate it into specific processes, such as report writing.
- Teach and model process skills tied to new applications, for example, write brief replies and make no personal attacks to create a safe environment for reflection and discussion.
- Ensure that users know that what they contribute to the blog is being read and is valued.
- Respect the nomadic nature of physicians' computer usage patterns. Provide wallet-sized ID cards that contain the physicians' user names and passwords so that they can use a blog on home, office, or hospital computers.
- Allow for self-organization (Zimmerman, Lindberg, and Plsek 1998). Encourage users to come up with ideas for new uses, rather than mandating a top-down strategy.

Figure 11.3: Potential Uses for Blogs in Healthcare Settings

- As a way to improve interdisciplinary collaboration and break down silos, for example, a department blog that encourages individual sections to collaborate
- As a project management tool to link participants who are geographically separated and do not see each other every day, for example, as a tool that keeps track of individual assignments and deadlines for an implementation task force
- As a training, virtual mentoring site to facilitate sharing of information that offers the possibility of real-time feedback, for example, as a way that a newly hired physician can keep in touch with a mentor, and that can provide knowledge management content that has helped other new recruits in the past
- As a repository of medical guidelines and best practices
- As an informal way to showcase cutting-edge therapies and programs, for example, as a site for posting results of clinical trials, especially those that have recruited patients from the community
- For virtual department or section meetings
- As a way to post agendas, meeting minutes, and reports, and as a response link to allow members who are unable to be physically present to contribute
- For survey dissemination and analysis of questions of interest to a section or department
- As a method to facilitate periodic reporting (for example, of volume, outcomes, goals, and attainment of objectives)
- As a link for senior hospital executives to obtain real-time input to issues affecting physicians' efficiency and effectiveness
- For the development of physician referral networks, with not only photos and contact information but also a live electronic link for asking questions and providing information
- As a communication channel to provide rapid updates, as in a local, regional, or national crisis with health implications
- For posting of information from aggregators to allow healthcare professionals to subscribe to information of interest, such as articles, national guidelines, and national and international news stories, without needing to log onto multiple Internet sites or receive a burdensome amount of e-mail

CONCLUSION

Blogs allow people who may be geographically disconnected to network and collaborate at times that are mutually convenient. The user-friendly search characteristics facilitate using a blog as a data repository. Blogs allow team members to find out what is happening without wasting their time playing telephone tag and thus help them implement new ideas in a timely fashion.

Through transparent engagement, blogs encourage healthcare professionals to share their thoughts and feelings, and blogs help create an environment from which new approaches may emerge because they lessen the risks of humiliation and failure. For complex organizations that acknowledge that innovation occurs at the edge of chaos (Cohn 2005), blogs allow people to try out new ideas and benefit from the collective intelligence of the group.

KEY CONCEPTS

- A blog is an Internet-based, user-friendly content management system useful for harried professionals seeking ways to make their time count, improve their practice environment, enhance physician-physician communication, and facilitate physician-hospital collaboration.
- Blogs make it easy for healthcare professionals to collaborate with colleagues at times of mutual convenience.
- Blogs mirror the way practicing physicians work: decentralized, searchable, and available 24/7.
- A proactive but flexible organizational policy regarding blog use that encourages informal communication and discourages leaks of proprietary information and patient health information is necessary to foster spontaneity and serendipity.

APPENDIX 11.1 WEB 2.0: LARGER IMPLICATIONS FOR BLOGS IN MEDICAL SETTINGS

Blogs and aggregators are two technologies making possible the evolution of the Internet from its historic use for centralized content distribution into a medium focused on people rather than content. The technology and philosophy behind this shift is collectively known as Web 2.0 (O'Reilly 2005). The Web 2.0 model recognizes that intelligence is distributed across a network of users and that in a world where knowledge is advancing so rapidly that innovation may come from many settings, it is more valuable to *connect with the person* who may be the source of useful information than to find static content.

Blogs have made it easy for anyone to publish for a wide audience on issues about which they are passionate. For example:

- Dr. Robert Centor's blog is called DB's Medical Rants (medrants.com); DB refers to his golfing nickname, "Da Boss." He writes, "As a generalist and internist, I'm disgusted with reimbursement.... This gives me a chance to talk about that" (Cook 2003).
- Dr. Penny Marchetti was an early adopter, starting Medpundit (medpundit.blogspot.com) in February 2002 to interpret medical news for her patients (Cook 2003).
- Shrinkette.blogspot.com comments on mental health news (Landro 2005).
- Thecheerfuloncologist.blogspot.com reflects the comments of a practicing oncologist (Landro 2005).
- Codeblog.com is a nurse's blog that encourages healthcare professionals to share stories and approaches to dealing with difficult patients (Landro 2005).
- Bioethicsdiscussion.blogspot.com, written by the chair of a community hospital ethics committee, invites comments on subjects such as end-of-life care and the place of religion and prayer in medicine (Landro 2005).

- Matthew Holt uses his blog to draw attention to healthcare policy articles and discuss Medicare, insurers, and electronic medical records, among other topics (*Wall Street Journal* 2005) (www.thehealthcareblog.com).
- On his blog Over My Med Body, a third-year medical student posted a Medicare Prescription Drug Calculator Tutorial, and posts a weekly "Grand Rounds" that includes the best of medical blogs across the Internet (http://www.grahamazon.com/2005/11/its-time-for-grand-rounds/) (*Wall Street Journal* 2005).

Using blogs, medical practitioners now have a vastly increased ability to share information and build networks across institutional boundaries with others who have similar interests. Institutions are beginning to recognize the value of blogs for harnessing the collective intelligence of their members.

- Dr. Marcus Pierson hopes to use his blog to revolutionize care for patients with chronic diseases. His hospital, St. Joseph Medical Center, is working with the Institute for Healthcare Improvement to involve the entire community in improving the healthcare system. He summarized his interest in using a blog by writing: "When you become a thinker about any business, including healthcare, the boundaries are completely porous—the system of healthcare involves everybody. **You need a medium to communicate that is not constrained by organizational boundaries**.... You try to have a technology to change the culture and a community by being open and telling stories ... to be able to get innovators in healthcare to get a place where we can work together across organizational lines" (Cook 2003).
- The American College of Surgeons acted on suggestions from the Residents and Associates Society and the Committee on Young Surgeons to develop a web-based

portal to improve relationships with members, simplify access to information, and build specialized virtual member communities (Russell 2004, Sheldon 2006).

- Children's Hospital of Seattle used a blog to complement its knowledge management system and assemble a searchable data repository of departmental policies and procedures (Ives and Watlington 2005, 121).

REFERENCES

Cohn, K.H. 2005. "Embracing Complexity," in *Better Communication for Better Care: Mastering Physician-Administrator Collaboration*, 30–38. Chicago: Health Administration Press.

Cohn, K.H. 2002. "The Structured Dialogue Process: A Successful Approach for Partnering with Physicians." *Click* [Online article; created 3/20/02.] www.acpe.org/Click

Cook, B. 2003. "Welcome to the Blogosphere: A Brave New World of Web Dialogue." [Online article; retrieved 10/1/2004.] http://www.mam-assn.org/amaednews/2003/04/28/bisa0428.htm.

Ives, B., and A.G. Watlington. 2005. *Business Blogs: A Practical Guide.* Charlestown, MA: Maranda Group.

Landro, L. 2005. "Net Benefits." *The Wall Street Journal* [Online article; retrieved 10/11/04.] http://online.wsj.com.article_email/article_printSB112854293262960833-MyQjAxMDE1.

Mohr, G. 2005. "All About Aggregators." [Podcast, retrieved 11/21/05.] http://learning2.o.ottergroup.com/blog/_archives/2005/11/17/1410673.html.

O'Reilly, T. 2005. *What is Web 2.0?* [Online Information.] http://www.oreillynet.com/pub/a/oreilly/tim/news/2005/09/30/what-is-web-20.html?page=2

Robeznieks, A. 2005. "Privacy Fear Factor Arises." *Modern Healthcare* 35 (46): 6–7,16.

Russell, T. 2004. "From My Perspective." *Bulletin of the American College of Surgeons* 89 (10): 3–4.

Sheldon, G.F. 2006. "Introducing e-facs.org: College Launches Web Portal for Its Members." *Bulletin of the American College of Surgeons* 90 (12): 12–16.

The Wall Street Journal. 2005. "What the In-Crowd Knows." *The Wall Street Journal*, November 16, D1.

Zimmerman, B., C. Lindberg, and P. Plsek. 1998. *Edgeware: Insights From Complexity Science for Health Care Leaders*. Irving, TX: VHA Inc.

CHAPTER 12

Collaborative Leadership at Academic Medical Centers

Kenneth H. Cohn, Carol Scott-Conner,
Keith Lewis, and Elaine Ullian

> I fear that if I lose my block time I will be unable to organize my schedule and balance my clinical and administrative responsibilities.... It just won't work."
> —*Surgeon during a discussion of proposed operating room*
> *changes*

INTRODUCTION

Academic medical centers (AMCs) are hospitals associated with medical schools and provide services traditionally not found in community hospitals, services such as transplantation, complex cardiac surgery, and care for patients who sustain life-threatening injuries requiring the collaboration of multiple services. Academic medical centers often have leading-edge technologies and drugs capable of dramatically altering traditional medical treatment. Over the last decade, many of the services traditionally performed only in AMCs have migrated to community hospitals, while sicker and more complex patients have remained behind.

Academic medical centers traditionally have a tripartite mission to provide patient care, perform cutting-edge laboratory and clinical research, and educate students, residents, postgraduate fellows, and allied healthcare professionals. Because of their mission of training healthcare professionals, AMCs are a place where trainees can learn communication and collaboration skills prior to entering practice. The purpose of this chapter is to highlight the expertise and leadership role of AMCs and the opportunity that an AMC has to influence the training of physicians and nurses who observe daily interactions between physicians, allied healthcare professionals, and administrators. The following case describes a way of boosting operating room (OR) efficiency through collaboration that may be relevant to other U.S. hospitals. The chapter concludes with a discussion of challenges facing AMCs and steps that may facilitate achieving their goals.

CASE PRESENTATION

Boston Medical Center, a 547-bed AMC affiliated with Boston University, faced a difficult challenge in 2003. Its emergency department (ED) was the busiest in Boston, averaging over 120,000 patient visits per year, but ambulances were diverted more than 20 hours per month to other hospitals because of capacity constraints (Reinert 2004). In addition, the bumping of elective surgical procedures by emergency cases made it difficult for patients, families, and surgeons to predict when surgery would actually occur, adding hours of nursing overtime to the existing budgetary stress and necessitating additional anesthesia coverage at later hours of the day and evening.

Dr. Eugene Litvak, director of the Program for Management of Health Care Variability at Boston University, analyzed data and suggested that smoothing the number of elective operations (spreading four to six procedures over the course of a week rather than booking all of them on one day of the week) and keeping one OR separate for emergencies might improve the situation. However, devoting one OR to emergencies meant that only seven

ORs would be available for elective cases. Hospital leaders faced the difficult task of persuading surgeons to try this radical idea, which required surgeons to relinquish block time.

Dr. Litvak stressed the importance of carefully controlling the booking of elective cases so that the hospital could avoid multiple patients simultaneously requiring ICU care postoperatively on a particular day. According to his recommendation, one OR was to be dedicated solely to emergencies, would not perform any elective cases, and would be fully staffed with anesthesia and nursing ready for patients from the ICU and ED who required emergent surgery. Cases requiring urgent surgery would be prioritized into different time categories based on how soon they required an operation: emergent (0 to 30 minutes), urgent (30 minutes to 4 hours), semi-urgent (4 to 24 hours), and non-urgent (greater than 24 hours). Creating these categories stressed the importance of the time from original diagnosis to surgical incision, avoiding potentially dangerous delays for patients because of inability to be placed on the OR schedule.

Hospital leaders persuaded the chief of vascular surgery to spread his cases over the entire week rather than performing elective surgery only on Wednesday and Thursday, which had created logjams in the ICU and step-down units and made it difficult for patients to be admitted from the ED to the patient-care floors. At the same time, cardiac surgeons changed their clinic days to spread their cases evenly from Monday through Friday.

At the same time that the urgent OR was created, block booking was eliminated and an open scheduling model was instituted, dedicating two ORs to orthopedics and making the remaining five ORs available to all other services for booking.

Creating an open urgent room and eliminating block booking resulted in a precipitous drop in the bumping of elective surgery from 349 to 7 cases during a similar timeframe before and after the creation of the open room (*OR Manager* 2004). Since initiating the open room in April 2003, only 9 patients as of December 2005 were bumped due to emergency cases, and the effort has received total buy-in and surgeon satisfaction because of the more efficient utilization of ORs during the day. Urgent cases are addressed in a timely manner rather than at the end of the elective schedule in the late afternoon or early evening. At the same time that bumping was nearly eliminated on this campus, surgical volume increased 3 percent after the elimination of block time.

Emergency department diversion hours dropped approximately 20 percent at Boston Medical Center even though the number of diversion hours in Boston as a whole increased 1.5 percent over the same time period (Stoddard 2004). The hospital changes decreased the average ED stay by 30 minutes (*OR Manager* 2004) by bringing patients into the rooms faster, streamlining their evaluation in the ED, and working with the bed coordinator to transfer admitted patients to the floors quickly following their evaluation. Although not directly measured, patient complaints decreased significantly with the near-total elimination of bumping of elective cases by emergency cases.

CASE ANALYSIS

Overcrowding was not a major issue until about 15 years ago when hospitals began reducing beds to decrease cost. However, aging demographics have increased demand steadily, causing capacity constraints and making inefficiency more apparent (Stoddard 2004).

Proposing an alternative to conventional scheduling, referred to as "operating outside the block," was an extremely difficult sell to surgeons because the hospital would need to take back operating time to create an available room for emergencies. Even though the burden was spread over all services and the impact on an individual surgeon was small, the perception was that this change would impose additional stress and hardship. Significant time and effort went into an educational campaign, and hospital leaders met with the busiest surgeons to ensure buy-in from all participants. The success of the changes described above reflected:

- the availability of an international expert who studied capacity constraints in other industries, applied them to healthcare in a data-driven fashion, and was able to demonstrate linkages between OR, ICU, and ED processes and outcomes,
- teamwork led by the chairmen of anesthesiology and surgery, who transcended departmental fiefdoms to improve the functioning of the larger system,
- confronting the facts prior to initiating process change by including all physician stakeholders to work out hidden agendas,
- the support of the CEO and chief medical officer, assuring constant review and modifications, with no operative cases refused, and
- a process of active communication at regular intervals that limited the power of rumor to interfere with proposed changes.

Open scheduling allowed surgeons to place cases on the elective schedule quickly, accommodated unpredictable volume surges for surgeons and services, and encouraged surgeons to schedule as early as possible. The traditional block-booking model may not accommodate volume variances between services and requires active and aggressive oversight to avoid large holes in the schedule when a service does not adequately use its block time.

CHALLENGES FACING AMCs

The challenges that AMCs face are related to the wide scope of their missions and to the funding challenges that all medical centers face in providing care for an increasing number of patients who are underinsured or uninsured.

Faculty Supervision

Faculty time seems to be spread more thinly due to the need to generate clinical revenue, be academically productive as reflected in publication in peer-reviewed journals, and teach students, residents, and fellows. The federally mandated 80-hour resident work week has decreased exposure to outpatient experiences (Spencer and Teitelbaum 2005) and limited continuity of care (Russell 2005). In the absence of strong systems of care, important details can fall through the cracks, threatening patient safety (Polk 2005).

Funding Uncertainty

Providing indigent care usually requires accepting reimbursement that falls below cost and arrives months after submitting bills. Because research funding tends to be for three-year periods, maintaining grant support is uncertain. Very few institutions have separate funding streams for medical school or residency teaching; the inequality of the legs of the three-legged stool funding patient care, research, and education increases faculty stress and creates instability in AMCs' business models.

Resistance to Change

AMCs tend to be loosely coupled, large institutions that receive input from multiple stakeholders whose allegiance tends to be toward departmental or sectional silos rather than to the institution as a whole. Without shared vision and collective energy, it is difficult for AMCs to achieve lasting reforms in a disruptive health-care marketplace (Souba 2004).

Technologic Advances

With the introduction of multiple new technologies and costly new designer drugs, AMCs are faced with challenges in deciding which new and advanced treatment options to provide to remain competitive and at the same time cost conscious. With new technologies such as robotic surgery and minimally invasive procedures, simulation may become an integral part of the AMC, so that medical students and residents can become proficient in necessary procedural skills prior to direct patient exposure (Greene et al. 2006).

New Aspects of Competition

The movement of many procedures from the OR to physician-owned outpatient facilities such as ambulatory surgical centers has created competition with the hospital (Cohn 2005) for orthopedic procedures, for example. Additional physician-physician turf battles, involving which specialty (cardiology, radiology, or vascular surgery) inserts endvascular stents, for example, have added complexity to decision-making processes.

LEADERSHIP AT ACADEMIC MEDICAL CENTERS

Souba (2004) wrote that leadership at AMCs needs redefinition. Previously, leadership centered on the achievements, contributions, and drive of a talented individual. However, leadership today needs to permeate all levels of an AMC. Only the collective energy of many people pursuing a common vision will allow AMCs to survive and thrive in the future. By focusing on coordinated teamwork, evidence-based care, and prevention of complications, as well as by learning and teaching communication skills, healthcare professionals can build high-quality connections and ensure long-term, sustainable success. They also can teach by example important lessons to their trainees.

Leadership is not only about the people in charge but also about building the transparency, trust, accountability, and collaboration that drive progress. Emotional intelligence, which requires leaders to be attuned to others' feelings (Goleman, Boyatzis, and McKee 2002), is a critical skill, because unlike finance and marketing, it cannot be delegated.

Evidence that clinical outcomes depend on teams may require changes in the training of healthcare professionals (Gawande 2001). McDade and colleagues (2004) reported that faculty scored significantly higher in leadership ability, including communication, networking, coalition-building, and conflict management, after completing the Executive Leadership in Academic Medicine (ELAM) program designed at their institution. Lee and colleagues (2004) developed a leadership training workshop for residents to build confidence in managing teams and leading group discussions. Awad et al. (2004) described a novel leadership curriculum designed to broaden residents' focus from a command-and-control approach toward a more collaborative approach by establishing specific objectives to meet the six core competencies that the Accreditation Council for Graduate Medical Education (ACGME) established for graduates of U.S. residency programs (Frey et al. 2003). The work of Frey, Lee (2004), and Awad (2004) and their colleagues is valuable because it uses validated survey methods to measure changes in knowledge and behavior that are difficult to evaluate objectively, especially for the last three ACGME competencies. The six competencies are as follows:

1. Compassionate, appropriate, and effective patient care
2. Medical knowledge about biomedical, clinical, and cognitive sciences
3. Practice-based learning and improvement
4. Interpersonal communication skills that result in effective information exchange
5. Professionalism
6. Awareness of systems of healthcare that transcend individual doctor-patient relationships

CONCLUSION

Academic medical centers can provide leadership in improving not only our understanding of molecular pathophysiology but also our ability to work together in complex systems to improve patient care. Developing new models of working together in the OR, as discussed in the case presentation, can have an impact on patients cared for at AMCs and on healthcare professionals in training who will leave AMCs to work in community facilities.

KEY CONCEPTS

- Academic Medical Centers (AMCs) are a unique and valuable resource on which the training of healthcare professionals depends.
- In addition to providing support to community hospitals for treatment of complex patients involving rare diseases or multiple comorbid conditions, AMCs also train future community hospital workers.
- Formal teaching of communication skills to medical students, residents, postgraduate fellows, nurses, and other allied healthcare professionals can benefit all types of hospitals in need of improved collaboration (these communication skills include empathic listening, win-win negotiation, conflict recognition and resolution, and leadership styles that go beyond command and control, as discussed in Chapter 7).
- With new technologies such as robotic surgery and minimally invasive procedures, simulation may become an integral part of the AMC, so that medical students and residents can become proficient in necessary procedural skills prior to direct patient exposure.
- Healthcare professionals must listen, understand, and meet the changing needs of patients and families on an ongoing basis and teach trainees to achieve outstanding clinical outcomes.

REFERENCES

Awad, S.S., B. Hayley, S.P. Fagan, D.H. Berger, and F.C. Brunicardi. 2004. "The Impact of a Novel Resident Leadership Training Program." *American Journal of Surgery* 188 (5): 481–84.

Cohn, K.H., and T.R. Allyn. 2005. "When Physicians Compete with the Hospital." *Better Communication for Better Care: Mastering Physician-Administrator Collaboration*. Chicago. Health Administration Press, 17–23.

Frey, K., F. Edwards, K. Altman, N. Spahr, and R.S. Gorman. 2003. "The 'Collaborative Care' Curriculum: An Educational Model Addressing Key ACGME Core Competencies in Primary Care Residency Training." *Medical Education*. 37 (9): 786–89.

Gawande, A.A. 2001. "Creating the Educated Surgeon in the 21st Century." *American Journal of Surgery* 181 (6): 551–55.

Goleman, D., R. Boyatzis, and A. McKee. 2002. *Primal Leadership: Realizing the Power of Emotional Intelligence*. Boston: Harvard Business School Press.

Greene, A.K., D. Zurakowski, M. Puder, and K. Thompson. 2006. "Determining the Need for Simulating Training of Invasive Procedures." *Advanced Health Science Education Theory Practice* 11 (1): 41–49.

Lee, M.T., A.M. Tse, and G.S. Nuguwa. 2004. "Building Leadership Skills in Paediatric Residents." *Medical Education* 38 (5): 545–76.

McDade, S.A, R.C. Richman, G.B. Jackson, and P.S. Monahan. 2004. "Effect of Participation in the Executive Leadership in Academic Medicine (ELAM) Program on Women Faculty's Perceived Leadership Capabilities." *Academic Medicine* 79 (4): 302–309.

OR Manager. 2004. "Boston Hospital Sees Big Impact from Smoothing Elective Schedule." *OR Manager* 20 (12): 1,10–12.

Polk, H.C. 2005. "Presidential Address: Quality, Safety, and Transparency." *Annals of Surgery* 242 (3): 293–301.

Reinert, S. 2004. "Hospital Experiment Cuts Wait for Patients." *The Patriot Ledger*. May 14, 1.

Russell, T.R. 2005. "Are 80 Hours a Week Enough to Train a Surgeon?" [Online article; retrieved 9/13/05.] http://www.medscape.com/viewarticle/511285.

Souba, W.W. 2004. "New Ways of Understanding and Accomplishing Leadership in Academic Medicine." *Journal of Surgical Research* 117 (2): 177–86.

Spencer, A.U., and D.H. Teitelbaum. 2005. "Impact of Work-Hour Restrictions on Residents' Operative Volume on a Subspecialty Surgical Service." *Journal of the American College of Surgeons* 200 (2): 670–76.

Stoddard, T. 2004. "BUMC Streamlines Emergency Care with Help from SMG Professor." *B.U. Bridge* 8 (8): 1–3.

Epilogue

This book is about changes in healthcare that provide hope for physicians, nurses, and hospital executives. Too often, we equate change with being asked to do more with fewer resources rather than as an opportunity to reflect, reframe our assumptions, and collaborate to achieve outcomes that we cannot accomplish on our own. The first three chapters on structured dialogue, creative abrasion, and hospitalists challenge widely held assumptions that healthcare professionals act principally out of self-interest and thus merit suspicion and careful supervision. The next six chapters on crew resource management, trends, adaptive design, leadership development, hospital design, and disease-based care offer field-tested strategies for boosting collaboration, safety, and satisfaction.

Physicians, nurses, and hospital executives all fear the clinical and economic consequences of the current malpractice climate. Chapter 10 examines malpractice as a failure of collaboration and outlines seven proactive steps that can decrease risk and improve outcomes.

The final chapters discuss the role of the Internet in building virtual communities of practice among healthcare professionals who do not have as much face-to-face contact as they did a decade ago and ways that academic medical centers can train future health-care professionals to think creatively and work interdependently to improve care.

Stubblefield (2005) wrote that people are our only hope for achieving true and lasting cultural change. The challenge for leaders is to create an environment that supports learning and team-work so that people have the freedom and support to do what they dreamed of when they began careers in healthcare. He acknowledged the role of passion that attracts people to health-care and empowers them to live out their dreams:

> "At times, we even have to revive that passion in employees who have allowed the daily frustrations and challenges of their jobs to overshadow their initial motivation. Everyone needs an occasional reminder that their work is about more than a paycheck, *that they are making a difference by doing what they do.*"

Building a culture of collaboration in healthcare supports learning and professional growth, allows people to take prudent risks, and makes it easier to deal with the conflict, dynamic change, and complexity that surround us. I hope that reading this book will stimulate discussion, energize people seeking change in their own and their patients' lives, and help dedicated professionals reconnect with the aspirations that attracted them to healthcare in the first place.

REFERENCE

Stubblefield, A. 2005. *The Baptist Health Care Journey to Excellence: Creating a Culture That WOWs!*, 40. Hoboken, NJ: John Wiley & Sons, Inc.

Suggested Reading

Atchison, T.A. 2006. *Leadership's Deeper Dimensions: Building Blocks to Superior Performance*. Chicago: Health Administration Press.

Brideau, L. 2004. "Flow: Why Does It Matter?" *Frontiers of Health Service Management* 20 (4): 47–50.

Cooperrider, D.L., D. Whitney, and J.M. Stavros. 2003. *Appreciative Inquiry Handbook*, 272. Bedford Heights, OH: Lakeshore Publishers.

Dorsey, D. 2000. "Positive Deviant." *Fast Company* 41 (December): 284. [Online article; retrieved 10/14/05.] http://pf.fastcompany.com/magazine/41/sternin.html.

Finkelstein, S. 2003. *Why Smart Executives Fail: And What You Can Learn from Their Mistakes*, 213–38. New York: Penguin Books.

Gill, S.L. 1987. "Can Doctors and Administrators Work Together?" *Physician Executive* 13 (5): 11–16.

Larson, L. 2002. "Balance of Power: Encouraging Physicians to Help Set the Strategic Plan." *Trustee* 55 (8): 12–17.

Ludema, J.D., D. Whitney, J. Bernard, and J. Thomas. 2003. *The Appreciative Inquiry Summit: A Practitioner's Guide for Leading Large-Group Change*. San Francisco: Berrett-Koehler.

Marcus, L.J., and B.C. Dorn. 2001. "Beyond the Malaise of American Medicine." *Journal of Medical Process Management* 16 (5): 227–30.

Miller, J.G. 2004. *QBQ: The Question Behind the Question*. New York: Putnam.

Patterson, K, J. Grenny, R. McMillan, and A. Switzler. 2005. *Crucial Confrontations*. New York: McGraw Hill.

Rosenberg, M.B. 2003. *Nonviolent Communication: A Language of Compassion*, 2nd ed. Encinitas, CA: Puddle Dancer Press.

Savary, L.M., and C. Crawford-Mason. 2006. *The Nun and the Bureaucrat: How They Found a Simple, Elegant Solution to a Deadly National Healthcare Problem*. Washington, DC: CC-M Productions, Inc.

Stubblefield, A. 2005. *The Baptist Health Care Journey to Excellence: Creating a Culture That WOWs!* Hoboken, NJ: John Wiley & Sons, Inc.

Studer, Q. *Hardwiring Excellence*. 2003. Gulf Breeze, FL: Fire Starter Publishing.

Tucker, A.L. and A.C. Edmondson. 2003. "Why Hospitals Don't Learn from Failures: Organizational and Psychological Dynamics that Inhibit System Change." *California Management Review* 45 (2): 55–72.

Ury, W.L. 1991. *Getting Past No*. New York: Bantam.

Zimmerman, B., C. Lindberg, and P. Plsek. 1998. *Edgeware: Insights from Complexity Science for Health Care Leaders*. Irving, TX: VHA Inc.

About the Author

Kenneth H. Cohn, M.D., MBA, FACS, is a board-certified general surgeon who obtained his M.D. degree from Columbia College of Physicians Medical School, completed his residency at the Harvard-Deaconess Surgical Service, and performed fellowships in endocrine and oncologic surgery at the Karolinska Hospital and at Memorial Sloan-Kettering Cancer Center at Brooklyn. He later moved to Dartmouth-Hitchcock Medical Center as associate professor of surgery and chief of surgical oncology at the VA Hospital at White River Junction.

With the change in the medical economic climate, Dr. Cohn entered the MBA program of the Tuck School at Dartmouth and graduated in June 1998. He worked initially as a consultant at Health Advances, assisting six firms to commercialize new products. Since joining the Cambridge Management Group, he has led change-management initiatives for physicians at affiliated hospitals within the Yale New Haven, Banner Colorado, Cottage Santa Barbara, and Sutter Sacramento Health Systems. Dr. Cohn remains clinically active, covering surgical practices in New Hampshire and Vermont.

Dr. Cohn's writing experience includes 38 published articles in peer-reviewed medical journals. His first book, *Better Communication for Better Care: Mastering Physician-Administration Collaboration*, was published by Health Administration Press in March 2005.

About the Contributors

Thomas R. Allyn, M.D., is the medical director and chief executive officer of the Santa Barbara and Lompoc Artificial Kidney Centers as well as the chief of nephrology and cochairman of the Medical Advisory Panel at Santa Barbara Cottage Hospital. He also serves on the adjunct USC faculty as an assistant clinical professor of medicine.

Jack Barker, Ph.D., is managing principal at Mach One Leadership, Inc., in Miami, Florida. A graduate of and former professor at the United States Air Force Academy, Dr. Barker received a doctorate in cognitive psychology at Florida State University. Dr. Barker is currently a pilot for United Airlines and has been called upon by healthcare organizations to present information about team dynamics and the aviation industry model for use in improving patient safety.

Murray F. Brennan, M.D., is chairman of the department of surgery at Memorial Sloan-Kettering Cancer Center in New York City, a position he has held for 20 years. Dr. Brennan was born and educated in New Zealand.

Carol Boswell, Ed.D., R.N., is an associate professor with Texas Tech University Health Sciences Center School of Nursing at the

Odessa, Texas, campus. She has published and presented in local, state, national, and international venues on topics related to health literacy, communication, education, leadership, research, and ethics.

Sharon Cannon, Ed.D., M.S.N., is regional dean and professor of nursing at Texas Tech University Health Sciences Center in Odessa, Texas.

C. Duane Dauner, FACHE, is president of the California Hospital Association in Sacramento. Mr. Dauner's association with hospitals began in 1966 when he became director of research at the Kansas Health Facilities Information Service. In 1968, he became vice president of the Kansas Hospital Association where he served until his appointment as president and chief executive officer of the Missouri Hospital Association in 1975. In 1985, Mr. Dauner was appointed president and CEO of the California Association of Hospitals and Health Systems (later to become the California Hospital Association).

James L. Dorsey, M.B.A., served four years as an academic medical center CFO and six years in an executive capacity with clinical laboratory and mental health providers. Since 1985, he has been associated with Cambridge Management Group, a healthcare management consulting firm, of which he is a co-founder. He is a graduate of Harvard College and Harvard Business School.

Andrew Feldman, J.D., attained both his undergraduate and legal degrees from the State University of New York at Buffalo. He is the founding partner of Feldman, Kieffer & Herman, LLP, which has four offices in New York State. For over 35 years he has counseled and defended professionals in all fields, particularly in the areas of healthcare and professional liability.

Robert B. Harrington, M.B.A., has been active in health services management consulting since 1975. In 1985 Mr. Harrington became associated with Cambridge Management Group, a healthcare management consulting firm, of which he is a co-founder. He is a graduate of Dartmouth College and the Harvard Business School.

Bill Ives, Ph. D., is an independent consultant and writer who has worked with Fortune 100 companies in knowledge management and learning for over 20 years. He is now focusing on business applications of Web 2.0 and recently published *Business Blogs: A Practical Guide.* Prior to consulting, Dr. Ives was a research associate at Harvard University exploring the effects of media on cognition after receiving his doctorate in educatonal psychology from the University of Toronto.

John W. Kenagy, M.P.A, M.D., Sc.D., has been a nurse assistant, vascular surgeon, healthcare executive, and visiting scholar at Harvard Business School. His research and experience has developed Adaptive Design,® a management methodology that develops new capability to adapt and improve the complex, dynamic, unpredictable work of healthcare. In addition, he is clinical associate professor of surgery at the University of Washington and director of Kenagy & Associates, LLC, in Cambridge, Massachusetts.

Keith P. Lewis, M.D., is chairman of the department of anesthesiology at Boston Medical Center.

Daniel Litten, M.D., is a graduate of University of Texas–Houston medical school. He previously was a healthcare consultant at McKinsey & Company, and is presently a private-practice hospitalist at Santa Barbara Cottage Hospital in California.

Jain Malkin is president of Jain Malkin Inc. in San Diego, California. She heads a healthcare interior architecture firm specializing in evidence-based design. Ms. Malkin is the author of several books on healthcare design and lectures globally on these topics. She has degrees in psychology and environmental design and serves on the board of The Center for Health Design.

Glen Mohr, Ed.M., is president of The Otter Group, a company that develops technology-enhanced corporate learning and communications programs and specializes in integrating "Web 2.0" services to support learning and innovation. Most recently his work has included running the Global Markets Innovation Program for Merrill Lynch. He received his master's of education from Harvard Graduate School of Education.

Andrew H. Nighswander, J.D., has been active in healthcare in both the public and private sectors for more than 30 years. He was an official with Boston Department of Health and Hospitals and a commissioner with the Massachusetts Rate Setting Commission. Prior to joining the Cambridge Management Group, he was a senior executive at the Lahey Clinic, a 450-physician multispecialty group practice. Mr. Nighswander is a graduate of Dartmouth College and the Columbia University School of Law.

Robert Reid, Ph.D., is director of medical affairs for the three-hospital Cottage Health System in Santa Barbara, California. He is an obstetrician-gynecologist by training and has served as chief of staff and member of the board of directors of the flagship Santa Barbara Cottage Hospital. He is a past president of the Santa Barbara County Medical Society and the California Medical Association.

Carol E.H. Scott-Conner, M.D. Ph.D., M.B.A., is professor of surgery at the University of Iowa Carver College of Medicine in Iowa City. She was head of the department of surgery at the University of Iowa Carver College of Medicine from 1995 through 2004. She is the author or coauthor of nine textbooks and monographs, with two more in production.

David L. Sundahl, Ph.D., was a visiting scholar at Harvard Business School, where he studied, consulted, and wrote on innovation and the creation of new growth business with organizations. Since joining Kenagy & Associates in 2002 he has gained hands-on experience in implementing adaptive systems in healthcare with hospitals and health systems. His doctorate is from Harvard University and he has taught at Harvard and in China.

Donald J. Thieme, M.B.A., is executive director of the Massachusetts Council of Community Hospitals in Braintree, Massachusetts. Mr. Thieme was the managing partner of a Healthcare Consulting Practice at Ernst and Young for over 20 years. He has taught at several colleges and Universities and is a frequent speaker on healthcare issues.

Elaine Ullian, M.P.H., is president and chief executive officer of Boston Medical Center, the largest safety net/academic medical center in New England. Mrs. Ullian has worked in healthcare for more than 30 years, and was the chief architect of the successful merger of the former City of Boston public hospital system with the former Boston University Hospital to create Boston Medical Center— the first public/private integration of its kind in this country.